FATAL AIRCRAFT ACCIDENTS

A Pathologist's Notebook

FATAL AIRCRAFT ACCIDENTS

A Pathologist's Notebook

S.K. Adaval

KNOWLEDGE WORLD

KW Publishers Pvt. Ltd.
New Delhi

KNOWLEDGE WORLD

A KW Publishers Book
www.kwpublishers.com

Published in India by

Kalpana Shukla
KW Publishers Pvt Ltd
5A/4A, Ansari Road, Daryaganj, New Delhi 110002
email: knowledgeworld@vsnl.net / online.kw@gmail.com

ISBN: 978-81-87966-77-7

Typeset by Black Innovation, New Delhi and printed at Raj Kamal Electric Press

To Sally, Rashmi, Bob & Mikul
with love

Contents

Preface

The purpose of this book is to highlight aspects of Aviation Accident Pathology that have implications for the investigation of fatal air crashes. In many developing countries, when a fatal aircraft accident occurs, a medical doctor is often detailed to conduct autopsies on the fatalities. Most often, forensic doctors are allotted this duty. Because aviation accident pathology is rarely covered in postgraduate study, such doctors are often inadequately equipped for the task.

The investigation of air crashes can move very quickly. Many disciplines (e.g. medical, technical, administrative) are involved in the investigation and their sole purpose is to determine the cause of death/accident as quickly as possible. Consequently, the importance of conducting meticulous autopsies, and the role of Aviation Accident Pathology, more generally, can take a backseat. The involved pathologist must be ready to assert himself in ways that call attention to the value of his discipline. This book provides information on many important facets of Aviation Accident Pathology that the author has acquired from three decades of experience in conducting such investigations in India.

The methods employed in investigating fatal and non-fatal aircraft accidents are basically the same. However, it is obviously easier to determine the cause of an accident when survivors are available. When there are no survivors, conclusions must be drawn through a process of deductive reasoning, based on a detailed examination of all available evidence connected with the air crash. Investigations are a collaborative effort involving a number of specialists and, in this effort, the aviation pathologist plays an important role. The appraisal of autopsy findings from a 'dead body' may be able to provide evidential support comparable to that from a 'dead machine'. A meticulous examination of human remains by a trained pathologist is an essential part of investigation and its value has been realised all over the world.

Although the meticulous examination of human remains is vital, it is inadequate if considered in the absence of knowledge about the medical history of the aircrew, environmental factors, structural damage to the aircraft and use/abuse of safety equipment. The study of positions of bodies, the condition of clothing, crash factors and the possibility of exposure to toxic substances is important to reconstruct the sequence of events and to obtain a reasonably vivid picture of the accident.

When pathologists are summoned to investigate a fatal air crash, they are confronted with problems like 'what to look for' and 'how to proceed'. Here, it is a matter of 'WHAT ONE KNOWS, ONE SEES'. The doctor who is not trained in this discipline often lists the injuries and puts the cause of death as 'multiple un-survivable injuries', and the chapter is closed for good! Pathologists who are thoroughly trained in this subject proceed more meticulously. Their plan includes the following activities:

(a) Proceeding to the scene of accident as quickly as possible.
(b) Familiarising themselves with the circumstances of the accident by interacting with other authorities.
(c) Studying the position of the bodies vis-à-vis the wreckage.
(d) Examining clothing for evidence of burns and contamination with toxic agents.
(e) Becoming familiar with safety equipment, such as ejection seats, seat belts, harness systems, type of aircraft involved, its flight profile, internal structure and seating arrangement etc.
(f) Conducting a meticulous autopsy and recording injuries peculiar to aviation, recurring themes of injury and their sequence.
(g) Differentiating between ante-mortem and post-mortem trauma.
(h) Subjecting the biological samples to histopathology and toxicological examination.

(i) Preparing a detailed report and discussing it with other investigating agencies.

The interaction of the pathologist with other groups will be extremely useful. A multi-linear approach is always ideal in ascertaining the cause of the air crash, which may be medical or non-medical. If no technical cause of accident is discovered, the mishap is often attributed to 'human failure' or 'pilot error'. In this situation, pathologists assume an important role, as they are often called upon to assess the possibility that the pilot suddenly became incapacitated. Insight into the intricacies of the discipline of Aviation Accident Pathology will enable them to do full justice to the confidence reposed in them by the investigating teams.

In addition to highlighting the role of Aviation Accident Pathology and its usefulness in investigating fatal air crashes, I have briefly outlined the administrative set-up for investigating civil and military aircraft accidents, the autopsy procedures for detecting trauma peculiar to aviation accidents and recurring themes of injury, and the procedures for reconstructing the events that occurred before, during and after the accident. Some basic information on applied aspects of toxicology is provided, especially in relation to carbon monoxide, alcohol and commonly used medications.

The text material has deliberately been limited so that pathologists can quickly brush up their knowledge before proceeding to conduct the investigation. It may also help them to make a checklist of their own by including some of the points detailed therein. I am sure that this effort on my part to highlight the role of Aviation Accident Pathology in investigation of fatal aircraft accidents will be found useful by those who suddenly face this onerous task when they are relatively unprepared.

Acknowledgements

The first person to whom I owe thanks and gratitude is Air Marshal (Retired) G.N. Kunzru of the Indian Air Force, who inducted me into the discipline of Aviation Accident Pathology. Starting from his patronage, which he bestowed in his capacity as Senior Advisor in Pathology, he continued to extend this support from further up the ladder as Director General, Armed Forces Medical Services (Indian Air Force).

Several colleagues have provided valuable information and advice in writing this book. I am especially grateful to Air Commodore (Retired) U.B. Mathur (Indian Air Force) who, as a colleague and friend, added academic backing and stability to the chapters on toxicology and bird strike. Many Heads of the Institute of Aerospace Medicine (Indian Air Force), Bangalore (India) have lent useful support and not hesitated in providing valuable advice/material as and when required. To them, I extend my grateful thanks.

I would also like to thank Jill Yang and Bob Wyer for their help in copy-editing previous versions of this book and their meticulous and painstaking efforts to make this book more readable.

And finally, I acknowledge the patient and loving support given by my wife Sally and reassuring encouragement from my daughter Rashmi. My gratitude to them is most sincere and heartfelt.

PART 1: PATHOLOGY

CHAPTER 1

DEVELOPMENT OF THE CONCEPT OF AVIATION ACCIDENT PATHOLOGY

Pathology in the literal sense is the study (*logos*) of suffering (*pathos*). This branch of biological science, thus deals with the nature of disease through the study of its causes, its progress and its effects, together with associated alterations of structure and function. If the term "Aviation Pathology" is viewed from this general perspective, it would have to include all possible areas of aviation stresses, including injuries, heat, gravitational forces, hypoxia and vibrations. Mason[1] has, however, narrowed the scope of this discipline, restricting it to "a comprehensive study of aviation fatalities whereby the medical history of the casualty and the findings at autopsy can be correlated with the environmental factors, the structural or other damage to the aircraft and the use or abuse of equipment so that a complete picture of the accident may be formed". Thus, the present chapter is devoted to Aviation Accident Pathology with special reference to fatal aircraft accident investigations.

In the earlier days of aviation, the flyer himself used to make the aircraft, fly it and investigate the mishaps, if any. There was hardly any contribution from technical and medical branches. Perhaps the first reported death due to powered heavier-than-air machines occurred in the United States where medical investigation assumed historical importance. The famous Wright brothers (Orville and Wilbur) were flying their powered machines as early as 1903. Performance of their machine improved to such an extent that in 1908 the US army decided to assess this aircraft for their use. While the US Army representative, Lieutenant Thomas Selfridge, was flying along with Orville Wright, the aircraft crashed. Although Orville Wright survived,

Lieutenant Selfridge died after being evacuated to a hospital. An autopsy report indicated that the cause of death was head injury, possibly due to falling on the head. Lieutenant Henry "Hap" Arnold of the US army, who was subsequently detailed to fly, donned his football helmet to protect his head, the logic being based on the unfortunate death of Lieutenant Selfridge. This apparently small effort on the part of Lieutenant Arnold communicates in a nutshell the whole concept of Aviation Accident Pathology. It underlines the philosophy behind this discipline, whose primary aim is the investigation of aircraft accidents, gathering of information from such events, and subsequent use of this knowledge in preventing similar mishaps in the future.

With occasional exceptions, the role of medical science in the investigation of fatal air crashes remained insignificant until the 1940s. In 1921, an autopsy conducted on the body of a pilot showed "tuberculosis of spine with hemorrhage in a cold abscess". This condition was given due consideration in the investigation of the crash in which the aircraft dived and caught fire.[2] In the 1930s, alcohol was considered to be a possible factor in a number of accidents. An RAF pilot, who was recovering from a leg injury, hired an aircraft, flew recklessly and crashed, thus raising questions about whether his leg injury interfered with his flying efficiency. In 1948, an attack of angina in a pilot was suspected to be the cause of accident, based on autopsy findings. Some enlightening articles on the subject from Gilson[3], Hass[4] and Teare[5] evoked limited response and the only improvement observed was the painstaking list of injuries compiled by various pathologists during autopsies of air-crash victims. However, there was no thorough and scientific correlation between the injuries encountered and crash factors. Consequently, the information that was so painstakingly compiled and stored often remained underutilised.

The role of medical considerations in flying during both World Wars was limited to the establishment of physical fitness standards for aircrew and the understanding of high altitude physiology. Nevertheless, interest was generated in hypoxia, carbon monoxide contamination of the cockpit and pilot fatigue.

In 1955, Armstrong and his colleagues published a historical report on the famous Comet air disasters.[6] Because this investigation proved to be a landmark in the history of Aviation Accident Pathology, a brief discussion of it is warranted. On the morning of 10 January 1954, a Comet airliner took off from the Rome airport for London with 35 passengers. Twenty-five minutes later, it broke up over the sea near Elba. Within four hours, 15 bodies were recovered from an area of 1¼ mile diameter and were autopsied by Prof. A. Fornari of Pisa. On the evening of 08 April 1954, another Comet aircraft with 21 passengers disappeared while flying from Rome to Cairo. By the next evening, 5 bodies were recovered from the sea near Naples and a sixth body was found 10 days later. Four of these bodies were autopsied by Dr. Donald Teare in England. By this time, the bodies had been in the water for a duration of about 22 hours, much of which was in daylight.

There were striking similarities in the injury patterns of both accidents. Out of 21 bodies, 9 were more or less naked, 5 were scantily clad and 7 were fully or well clothed. The well-clothed bodies were of those passengers who had occupied the rearmost seats in each aircraft.

Out of 19 bodies studied, 14 had ante-mortem fractures of the skull and 15 had similar injuries to the thoracic cage. Fractures of extremities that were seen in 13 cases, appeared to have been caused after the cessation of circulation as they were bloodless. Internal injuries were extensive and occurred even in bodies showing minimal external trauma. Extensive lung damage was seen in all cases, with hemothorax in most of them. The lung injuries were deep and diffuse, occurring mostly in the lower lobes, with haemorrhagic margins and sub-pleural haemorrhages. There were contusions, lacerations, formation of sub-pleural bullae. No rib-marking was seen in any case. Histologically, traumatic emphysema was seen and fat embolism was found in 12 cases. Abdominal injuries were less frequent although hemoperitoneum and lacerations of the liver were common. Ruptured hearts were found in 4 cases, torn great vessels in 13, while hepatic lacerations was seen in all. Fourteen bodies of the Elba accident had areas of altered skin appearance like scalding, and 4 bodies of the Naples accident had patchy, pigmented appearance of the skin in some parts.

As the wreckage of the aircraft was still being searched, attention was focused on these findings. Although this situation had arisen by chance, it became instrumental in highlighting the medical aspects of air-crash investigation. Medical inquiry attempted not only to record all lesions encountered and to identify the cause of death but also to determine the sequence of events that led to the crash and the occurrence of the injuries. To attain this objective, the causes of pulmonary damage and skin pigmentation had to be specially established and ante-mortem injuries had to be segregated from immediate post-mortem trauma. Elaborate investigations were carried out at the Royal Aircraft Establishment in the United Kingdom. Full-scale clothed dummies were dropped in the sea to study the effect of impact on water. Anaesthetised guinea pigs were projected from a vertical catapult to approximate proper terminal velocities, and the injury pattern that occurred was studied.

Pulmonary damage consisted of congestion, contusions, lacerations, pulping and formation of sub-pleural bullae. Most of the lacerations had haemorrhagic margins and haemorrhagic sub-pleural zones extended deep into lung parenchyma without conforming to a 'rib-marking' pattern. Histologically, traumatic emphysema, congestion and haemorrhages were seen. Fat emboli were present in 12 cases.

For lung injuries, three possibilities were considered: blast, explosive decompression and severe impact (abrupt deceleration). Animal experiments with rabbits on "blast changes" showed bloody froth in the upper respiratory passages, visceral pleural haemorrhages and rib markings beneath intercostal spaces. This condition, known as concussion of lungs, was due to: (a) direct deformation of lung tissue, (b) differential acceleration of different structural elements and (c) chest wall flinging inwards at 20 metres/sec in 1/2 millisecond. In the Comet fatalities, there were no rib markings or bloody froth in respiratory passages. There were no burns or skin wounds due to flying missiles. External injuries were more or less similar in all bodies. In the event of a blast, persons sitting near the source of the blast are likely to be more severely affected. Consequently, this cause was ruled out, leaving explosive decompression and abrupt deceleration as possibilities.

Other evidence called the possibility of explosive decompression into question. As lungs have very high tolerance to explosive decompression, such injuries are possible only if the intensity of explosive decompression crosses certain limits and a minimum area of 290 sq. ft is lost in .032 seconds. This was considered very unlikely. (Later on, the wreckage showed that although an area of 162 sq. ft had been lost, the splitting process had been quite prolonged.) There was no gross air embolism or mediastinal emphysema, which is characteristic of explosive decompression. Therefore, this possibility was also unlikely.

Finally, the findings of animal experimentation (e.g. impacting guinea pigs on a water surface) established that such injuries were possibly due to abrupt deceleration. Similarly, internal injuries could also be attributable to impact on water, explaining how internal injuries can be extensive without significant external trauma. Experiments with dropping clothed dummies on a water surface from various altitudes showed that loss of clothing can also result from impact with water.

Skin changes observed in 14 of 15 bodies from the first accident comprised reddish irregular areas, especially under the clothing, without scorching or singeing of hair. Histologically, the epidermis in some areas was intact, whereas it separated or was absent in others. Epidermal cells showed vacuolar changes and accumulation of brown pigment in basal cells of 4 of the 5 specimens taken from fair European bodies. The dermis showed coagulative changes. The possibility of contact with hot metals, liquids or vapours in the aircraft, abrasion on impact, exposure to high-intensity flash, fall through flames and chemical burning were considered and ruled out. It was suggested on the basis of certain experiments that a film of kerosene burning on the water surface heated up the water sufficiently to cause such "scalds" in the bodies just underneath the water surface. Areas of darkened skin, encountered in 3 bodies of the Naples accident, were seen on exposed parts with sharp contrast to covered areas. The possibility of colouring with exogenous material or formation of a new pigment was ruled out and experiments suggested that darkening could have occurred due to enhancement of natural skin pigment by exposure to sunlight even after death, known as the Meirowsky Phenomenon.

A reconstruction of this accident, therefore, established that the injuries occurred in three different phases: in the aircraft, on impact with water and while in the water. Ante-mortem fractures of the skull could not have occurred by impact on water, as indicated by previous records in similar situations. They were, therefore, thought to be due to violent, upward and forward displacement of bodies at the time of cabin pressurisation failure. This failure could have caused fat embolism as well. Internal injuries could not have occurred during this phase, however. Rather, these injuries resulted from the bodies' spilling from the aircraft and impacting on the sea, which also caused the loss of clothing. Skin changes in the Elba accident could have been due to scalding water which was heated due to burning kerosene. In the Naples accident, however, accentuation of skin pigment resulted from exposure to the sun.

Establishment of Investigative Centres

Publication of the Comet findings conclusively proved the usefulness of Aviation Accident Pathology and its role in reconstruction of the events even when the wreckage was not immediately available. The findings of this investigation led to the establishment of the Department of Aviation Pathology in 1955 at the RAF Institute of Pathology and Tropical Medicine, based on the recommendations from two consultants in Pathology and Aviation Physiology, Air Commodore W.P. Stamm and W.K. Stewart. J.K. Mason was in charge of this department in the late 1950s and demonstrated the usefulness of this discipline in accident investigation. The channels of investigation he recommended[1] were:

(a) A study of the causes/modes of death in aircraft accidents with special emphasis on conditions peculiar to severe trauma and to aviation.
(b) Identification of the medical causes of accidents due either to internal or environmental abnormalities, and
(c) The reconstruction of obscure accidents by means of detailed examination of human remains.

In 1954, Wing Commander Bruce Harvey, an RAF physician stationed in Washington, had written a letter to Brig. Gen. Elbert Decoursey, Director of the Armed Forces Institute of Pathology (AFIP). It is interesting to recall a paragraph from this letter (Reals[7]):

"As you know, when a fatal accident occurs, engineers immediately descend upon the wreckage and take numerous samples back to their laboratories for investigation. The human remains, however, are usually collected together and put into a box and buried with due ceremony. May not the examination of such remains by a skilled pathologist provide evidence which may account for the accident?"

Subsequently, a conference was held under the Chairmanship of Wing Commander Harvey in 1955, comprising representatives from the US Army, Navy and Air Force, the AFIP, Cornell, Guggenheim Aviation Safety Center, National Institute of Health, Royal Navy, Royal Air Force and Royal Canadian Air Force. The conference recommended the formation of a committee on aviation pathology consisting of representatives from the USA, UK and Canada and another committee of pathologists at the Armed Forces Institute of Pathology (AFIP) to study the air-crash findings in depth and recommend various procedures for such investigations. An annual symposium and a new classification of air-crash etiology were also recommended. This conference strongly recommended that an autopsy be performed on every aircrew fatality. The Joint Committee on Aviation Pathology (JCAP) emerged from this historic conference.

The AFIP, Washington acted as the central coordinating body for investigating fatal aircraft accidents. An aviation pathology section was started and combined with the already functioning department of forensic pathology. In 1959, however, a new division known as Military Environmental Pathology Division was established, with Aerospace Pathology and Forensic Pathology as its branches. In 1956, facilities of toxicological investigations were created in the Aerospace Pathology branch. The Office of the Armed Forces Medical Examiner (OAFME) at AFIP in Washington DC is the JCAP Headquarters. This is the central coordinating facility for the investigation of human pathology from aircraft accident fatalities.[8]

Since then, the scientific literature on Aviation Accident Pathology has been enriched by pioneer workers from both the United States (e.g. KF

Mostofi, Webb Haymaker, Frank Hartman, Frank Townsend, Thaddeus Domanski, Leo Goldbaum, Frank Kiel, J. Gordon Webster, Warren Lovell, W.M. Silliphant, V.A. Stembridge, W.H. Davidson, W.J. Reals, S.R. Mohler and W.M. Glantz) and the United Kingdom (Air Vice Marshal W.J. Stamm, Group Captain J.K. Mason and P.J. Stevens).

Aviation Pathology services in Canada[9] and Australia developed along similar lines. The German Air Force established a department of aviation pathology at Fursten Feldbuck. In India, the idea of starting an aviation pathology cell was mooted in 1957 through a discussion between Group Captain S.P. Bhatia, Director Medical Services, Indian Air Force and Wing Commander M.M. Shrinagesh, his deputy. The cell started functioning at the Armed Forces Medical College (AFMC), Pune on 19 October 1959. A memorandum indicating a plan to study certain problems in Aviation Pathology was prepared by Wing Commander A.K. Basu, the first aviation pathologist posted to the cell. Procedures for medical investigation of fatal aircraft accidents were formulated under the guidance of Colonel P.N. Bardhan, Professor of Pathology, AFMC, Pune. This aviation pathology cell conducted examinations of biological samples from all fatal aircraft accidents of the Armed Forces on a centralised basis. Autopsies were generally performed by the pathologists available at peripheral hospital laboratories as a single aviation pathologist alone could not cover the vast zones. However, all histological and toxicological investigations were centred at this cell and autopsy reports were correlated with crash factors. In 1968, this cell was shifted to the Air Force School of Aviation Medicine, Bangalore. This school was subsequently upgraded to the status of an Institute. A Department of Aviation Toxicology was added in 1971.

Since 1958, an awareness of the usefulness of this discipline of Pathology has prevailed in all countries and attempts are being made to organise such establishments. The JCAP now holds regular scientific sessions and issues useful bulletins, which act as guidelines for a large number of medical investigators.

In 1961, a Ministry of Aviation Committee Report in the UK acknowledged the potential value of aeromedical specialists attending accident sites, in assessment of safety factors and cause of accident. The help of aviation pathologists from the RAF was sought in some accidents, among which the air crash involving the death of Mr. Dag Hammarskjold, Secretary General, UN, is notable. In 1963, Tweedie emphasised the role of aeromedical experts in fatal air-crash investigations. In the UK, it is now a routine practice for an Accident Investigation Branch (AIB) team to include a pathologist from the RAF Department of Aviation Pathology in all fatal aircraft accident investigations and no investigation of a fatal aircraft accident is considered complete if an autopsy has not been carried out.

CHAPTER 2

AVIATION ACCIDENT PATHOLOGY AND THE PATHOLOGIST

The main aim of any air-crash investigation (fatal or non-fatal) is to ascertain the factors that are responsible for the mishap. The factors could be human, material or environmental, and could have contributed directly or indirectly to the accident. If these factors can be identified, remedial measures might be undertaken to prevent such occurrences in the future. Preventive measures may entail proper selection procedures, improvement of environmental factors, safety equipment and even design of the aircraft.

During the operation of an aircraft, man and machine perform in an integrated manner. In the case of a fatal accident, therefore, it is unwise to ignore the man's body and concentrate only on technical aspects of the machine. On several occasions, the human body has provided better clues to determine the cause of accident than has the machine. To quote an example, the presence of ante-mortem burns on the body of a pilot can distinguish an in-flight fire from a post-crash conflagration. Similarly, the presence of haemorrhagic and bloodless fractures in the same body will enable an investigator to differentiate between injuries that occurred before the crash from those which resulted from a terminal massive impact. Such clear delineations are not always possible on the basis of technical evidence alone.[10–12]

In 1958, Townsend and Stembridge[13] showed that, despite best efforts, 14 per cent of all aircraft accidents in the USAF remained unexplained. In the case of fatal accidents, however, the percentage was 40. These figures show beyond doubt that in the absence of survivors, the cause of an accident is more difficult to determine.

As the trauma sustained during aviation is unique, the pathologist has to be fully conversant with such injuries. He must correlate his findings with those of other investigators who are experts in other disciplines of medicine and technology. According to Silliphant and Stembridge,[14] the work of a pathologist in such situations must deviate from the time-honoured routine procedures. Therefore, special training is necessary to inculcate an awareness of a multi-factorial 'man–aircraft' relationship. Niess et al.[15] have discussed the key contribution that the medical profession can make towards the promotion of flight safety. They have highlighted the importance of careful planning and involvement of pathologists and toxicologists in such an endeavour. Mason[1] emphasizes that the pathologist's main contribution lies in the assessment of safety equipment, which might have been either used or abused. The concept of full medical coverage of fatal aircraft accidents is widely acknowledged (Editorial, *British Medical Journal*[16]). The contribution of such coverage is basically flight-safety oriented.

As an aviation pathologist cannot work in isolation during the investigation of an accident, Platt and Townsend[17] highlight the need for an organised approach to aviation disasters. Mason[1] fully discusses the importance of teamwork in such investigations wherein the role of law, medico-legal authorities, engineers, doctors, flight safety workers and international bodies has been described and cooperation of research laboratories is highlighted. According to Mason and Tarlton,[18] a multi-linear approach to investigation implies the coordinated, yet independent investigation of an accident along circumstantial, engineering and medical dimensions. Gable[19] has discussed the value of certain injury patterns as pointers to medical investigators so that they can sequence the events. Adaval et al.[12] pointed out the setback that an investigation can receive when the services of a trained pathologist are not available for autopsies on air-crash victims. Townsend has highlighted medical aspects of aircraft accidents and the role of pathology in the investigation.[20,21] Berry's article on aircraft accident prevention is also worth mentioning.[22] Cullen et al.[23] have evaluated medical factors in 1,000 fatal aviation accidents. Adaval[24] has further highlighted the contribution of pathologists in such investigations, bringing into focus some aspects of traumatic pathology which, although obvious, are often overlooked by inexperienced forensic pathologists.

According to Kunzru et al.,[25] aviation pathologists should direct their investigations to the following main objectives:

(a) A reconstruction of the sequence of events surrounding the accident, with special attention to the possibility of survival;
(b) An appraisal of the use or abuse of safety equipment, and
(c) Discovery of the cause of accident (which may be medical or non-medical).

An ideal Aviation Pathology Investigation should essentially include the following steps (IAP No. 4305,1978)[26]:

(a) The pathologist should thoroughly familiarise himself with the type of aircraft involved in the accident, its internal structure, cockpit, seating arrangements, ejection mechanism, life support system, etc. It would be ideal to see an intact aircraft of the same type for this purpose.
(b) The pathologist should become properly acquainted with all available information on the circumstances of the crash and all relevant details of the aircrew, including their health and history of recent illness, if any.
(c) Careful observation and recording of crash-site findings pertaining to the positions of bodies vis-à-vis the wreckage, the state of clothing, life support systems, etc.
(d) A comprehensive autopsy, which should include histological and toxicological investigations.
(e) The correlation of autopsy findings with the medical history of the aircrew and relevant details of the accident that have been worked out by other investigating agencies.
(f) The submission of a comprehensive aviation pathology report to the concerned authorities.

Plan of Investigation

The role of Aviation Accident Pathology is essentially preventive. This discipline involves a very thorough investigation of fatal aircraft accidents, so that the knowledgegained can be utilised in the prevention of a recurrence.[3] A practical application of this principle is described by Mason[1] in his definition of Aviation Accident Pathology, which necessitates a "comprehensive" study of aviation fatalities. Whenever a fatal crash occurs, the medical evidence usually available is the human body and its medical history. This evidence is further linked to environmental factors, structural and other damage to the aircraft, and the use or abuse of safety equipment. This plan, which has been found to be very useful, is briefly summarised below:

I. Medical Factors

A. Medical History

1. Medical conditions which could cause sudden incapacitation/ limitation.
2. Surgical conditions hindering the ability to meet sudden requirements during an emergency.

B. Autopsy Findings

1. Gross autopsy findings
   - a. Trauma peculiar to aviation
   - b. Recurring themes of injuries
   - c. Evidence of survival during/after the crash
   - d. Differentiation between ante-mortem and post-mortem injuries
   - e. Evidence of pre-existing disease
   - f. Radiological support
2. Histopathological findings:
   - a. Traumatic histopathology
   - b. Sequencing of injuries
   - c. Evidence of survival after the crash
   - d. Sifting of ante-mortem and post-mortem trauma
   - e. Pre-existing diseases
3. Toxicological findings:
   - a. Carboxy-haemoglobin
   - b. Alcohol
   - c. Lactic acid
   - d. Drugs
   - e. Other toxic substances

II. **Environmental Factors** (Townsend and Stembridge,[13] Townsend [21,27,28])
   A. Altitude — to assess hypoxia, decompression
   B. Speed — to assess 'g' forces, spatial disorientation, windblast effect
   C. Toxic products — carbon monoxide, fuels, odours, chemicals
   D. Temperature — excessive heat, cold and humidity
   E. Noise — auditory effects, vibrations
   F. Stress — pathology of stress and fear

III. **Structural Damage to Aircraft**
   A. Pre-crash damage
   B. Post-crash damage

IV. **Safety Equipment**
   A. Crash helmet
   B. Flying clothing
   C. Oxygen system
   D. Survival pack

V. **Escape**
   A. Ejection seat
   B. Parachute

It is evident from the above that relevant information can be obtained from a comprehensive autopsy with background knowledge of the medical history of the deceased. Once this is done, the information can be correlated with environmental and other factors that are identified by specialists in other areas. To quote an example: a medical history of previous episodes of Ischemic Heart Disease, along with gross narrowing of coronary arteries discovered during autopsy (and confirmed histologically), may be relevant if the aircraft sustained sudden high 'g' forces with an unprotected pilot.[29] Thus, the medical history of the deceased and autopsy are two essential facets of medical investigation as far as the pathologist is concerned. These facets are discussed briefly in the following paragraphs.

A large number of conditions can cause the sudden incapacitation of a pilot. Some, which may bring about episodic unconsciousness in an apparently normal individual, are mentioned below:

1. Reduced blood supply to the brain (circulatory syncope)
   (a) Peripheral circulatory collapse
   (b) Vaso-vagal syncope
   (c) Postural hypotension
   (d) Effect of 'Gravitational Force (G)'
   (e) Tussive causes, e.g. breath-holding, valsalva, pressure breathing and coughing bouts
   (f) Drugs, esp. vasodilators, hypotensives and alcohol
   (g) Carotid sinus syndrome
   (h) Acute coronary episode[30,31]
2. Metabolic
   (a) Hypoxia
   (b) Hyperventilation
   (c) Hypoglycaemia
3. Cerebral
   (a) Epilepsy — idiopathic/symptomatic/atypical
   (b) Cerebral lesions — e.g. Berry's aneurysm
   (c) Colloid cyst of 3rd ventricle
4. Psychosomatic
   (a) Anxiety, panic, fear, etc.
   (b) Hyperventilation
5. Mixed
   (a) Combined effects of hypoxia, extremes of temperature, hypoglycaemia
   (b) Combined effects of 'g' loads with hyperventilation
   (c) Combined effects of sensitive carotid sinus with pressure breathing.

CHAPTER 3

AUTOPSY

The autopsy examination must be carried out as soon as possible. Delay can lead to the decomposition of bodies, resulting in the likely loss of valuable evidence. Many aircraft accidents occur at unpredictable and not easily accessible places. In such circumstances, it becomes difficult to get the body/bodies of victims removed to a proper mortuary and autopsy room within a reasonable period of time. This unavoidable delay has often led to the loss of valuable clues. Therefore, a change in the concept of an autopsy was inevitable. With this changed concept, the autopsy is taken to the body rather than taking the body for autopsy.

For practical application of this changed concept, certain essential facilities have to be created.

1. A state of readiness on the part of the pathologists along with their assistants so that they can proceed to accident site immediately.
2. Administrative authorities have to be briefed on such eventualities so that they can provide necessary information to the pathologists immediately after the crash and give them authority to move, without any procedural delay.
3. Mode of conveyance: This has to be the fastest possible under the prevailing circumstances. An ideal mode is by helicopter, which should be kept ready to fly the pathologist's team to the place of accident.
4. Equipment: As the autopsy may be performed on the spot, a portable autopsy kit is essential and should be kept ready at all times. This kit occupies minimum space, is lightweight and contains all essential equipment for an autopsy. It also contains photographic equipment,

sample collection containers along with preservatives, a portable autopsy table, autopsy instruments, a recording device to record the findings and a checklist of 'dos and don'ts'. Essential features of this 'Portable Autopsy Kit' are given in Chapter 9. In the absence of a ready-made autopsy kit, a pathologist can make one's own portable kit with the help of local authorities and keep it ready for such eventualities.

Autopsies must be performed on all deceased aircrew members who may have been involved in the actual operation of the aircraft or in essential flight activities. In the case of a passenger aircraft, autopsies must be performed on all casualties aboard the aircraft, irrespective of their numbers. It is advisable to use liberal photographic cover during such an investigation.[32] This helps to identify all deceased occupants of the crashed aircraft, which is essentially required on ethical as well as legal grounds. Moreover, the pattern of injuries sustained by passengers, along with the exact manner and cause of death of each, helps to reconstruct the pre-crash sequence of events. In addition, it can provide valuable information regarding passenger seating and safety equipment, leading to clues regarding the cause of accident. After identifying the casualties, for example, it is possible to consult the seat-chart and assign them to their respective seats. If the injury pattern shows that casualties were subjected to blast injuries and this finding was limited to only a few bodies grouped in a particular area of the aircraft, then the pathologist can provide reasonable evidence that the blast occurred at a particular place. This topic will be highlighted in detail when we consider injury analysis vis-à-vis autopsies.

After a detailed examination of the crash site and wreckage and making a photographic record of the crash (including positions of the bodies, state of safety equipment, etc.), bodies may be shifted to a suitable mortuary. If this is not feasible, any suitable building with a few essential facilities (e.g. light, running water and improvised tables) can be converted into a make-shift mortuary. Even in the absence of such facilities, however, it is worthwhile to carry out autopsies with whatever resources are available at the site of accident. (Under such circumstances, the portable autopsy equipment is invaluable.)

Before conducting autopsies and making an on-the-spot investigation, the pathologist will require some necessary information in order to evaluate autopsy findings in relation to the circumstances of the accident. Such information falls into three categories:

1. *Information about the aircrew*, including their age, past medical history, recent illnesses, training and experience, amount of stress and mental state, available flying aids, and the availability of supporting protective and safety equipment.
2. *Information about the mission*, including the flight profile, time of take-off, the type of sortie, the time of the crash, the weather, terrain and visibility, pre-crash flight factors such as 'g' effects, hypoxia and other flying stresses.
3. *Information about the machine*, including performance capabilities, cockpit conditions, and other peculiarities of the type of aircraft.

Besides the above, the pathologist should visit the crash site so that he can have a general idea about the crash site, wreckage, evidence of fire, impact angle, impact marks on the ground and position of body/bodies vis-à-vis wreckage. He should ask permission to examine protective clothing, safety equipment, ejection seat, etc. where applicable. In a passenger aircraft, the state of lap-belts, clothing of casualties and positions of the bodies in and outside the cockpit are of special significance.

Aim of the Autopsy

Conducting a post-mortem examination on all casualties in aircraft accidents has two objectives: (a) to evaluate the effect of environmental stress of flight on the individual, and (b) to establish the causative agent for the crash and the injuries, thus permitting the sequence of events to be reconstructed in relation to ante-mortem and post-mortem injuries. In addition, the examination can help to identify pre-existing factors that may have led the aircrew to become incapacitated.

The autopsy should be complete and thorough, regardless of any putrefaction, gross mutilation or disfigurement that results from post-crash factors such as fire. A high degree of suspicion, a skeptical mind, a tendency to avoid premature conclusions and a capacity for deductive reasoning are essential prerequisites for an aviation pathologist. He should stay calm and not be susceptible to pressure from administrative authorities, who often ask for very expeditious results and urge the conclusion of the investigation. These authorities can also try and bias the pathologist with their own theories about the cause of the accident. The pathologist should tactfully deal with such situations. Many times, an autopsy is discouraged by administrative as well as medical authorities due to paucity and mutilation of body parts. It is the duty of the pathologist to convince these authorities that in spite of fragmentation of body parts, a detailed examination of such remains may yield useful information.

Hellerich and Pollak[33] have highlighted this fact. They carried out a detailed study of fragmented pieces pertaining to six casualties from a one-engine light aircraft that struck ground at a high terminal velocity. They found detachment of skin with typically sharp-edged margins and striae-like tears due to over-stretching, intra-cutaneous haemorrhages conforming to pleats of clothing, thin-layer haemorrhages under articular cartilages, petechae of conjunctival serous membranes and mucous membranes of trachea and larynx. Separation of the penis with detachment of its skin and hematoma of glans/prepuce were seen whereas long peripheral nerves were well preserved due to their resistance to tearing. All these haemorrhages were thought to be of a local nature, as it was reasonable to assume that circulation of blood ceased on impact. These useful findings would have been lost if the tissue had not been examined.

Autopsy Procedure

Photography before the autopsy

A comprehensive photographic cover is of utmost importance. This can be provided by: (a) the Flight Surgeon, (b) the Squadron Medical Officer of Air Force, (c) a civilian doctor detailed by Director General of Civil Aviation (in India), or a Defence doctor who specialises in aviation medicine. The designated pathologist may not be the first to reach the scene of accident. In this case, a medical doctor (other than pathologist) should take on this responsibility. In the rush of things, vital evidence is often missed, disturbed or even ignored. Therefore, because it is later difficult to reconstruct such evidence from memory, the importance of photography is increased.

Photographs of undisturbed wreckage, bodies, life-support system, cockpit, gouge marks on the ground and nearby tree stumps should be taken from all necessary angles. Special attention should be paid to the relative position of each body vis-à-vis the wreckage. If possible, aerial views of the crash site should also be taken. Careful examination of the wreckage may reveal traces of human remains that should be photographed and labelled. The personal equipment of the victims and tears in their clothing may be necessary to supplement autopsy findings. Damage to helmets, oxygen equipment, harnesses and other safety equipment is also important to photograph without disturbing the fasteners, locks and buckles, etc.

Before an autopsy, the body should be carefully examined with all clothing on to allow a critical assessment of the clothing worn. Tears, stains, burns and presence of any foreign objects (including chemicals) should be noted and the exact place of their location on the clothing should be recorded. This information may later be correlated with underlying injuries to the body. The liberal use of photographic cover would help in this regard.[32] Personal equipment that may accompany the body should be appraised. Any evidence of fire is vital. Guidelines for autopsy photography have been laid down by OAFME.[34] All bodies must be photographed from anterior, posterior, lateral and oblique aspects. Helmets, personal effects and clothing should be labelled after photography. An autopsy number and a ruler/scale should be visible in each picture.

After removal of clothing, the body should be photographed from all angles and positive findings, if any, should be highlighted. This should be followed by complete X-ray of the body regardless of the paucity of human remains. This procedure is often considered to be wasteful. However, many fractures that are otherwise hard to detect can be seen on these X-rays. Evidence of shrapnel and other metallic objects can provide valuable clues concerning the likelihood of a blast or explosion. Whole-body X-rays with emphasis on head, neck, hands, feet and spine are recommended. In the case of pilots/co-pilots, X-rays of hands should be taken in detail to analyze 'control injuries' later on. In the case of fatal ejections, lateral views of occipital-first cervical junction with head, under 25 pounds of traction are required.[35]

A suitable plastic or paper bag, properly labelled, should be kept ready for each victim so that all personal effects, clothing, shoes and other items can be placed in the bag and sealed. Before beginning an autopsy, the pathologist should ensure that all necessary containers and preservatives are ready for blood, biological samples, and tissue that will be subjected to chemical and histological examinations.

Plan of the autopsy:

It is advisable to make a set plan while conducting the autopsy. Whereas some pathologists start recording the findings in a head-to-foot sequence, others go by external appearance, internal organs and skeletal system sequence. For the sake of convenience, some guidelines for identifying important injuries and their significance are mentioned below:

External Appearance

Note all external injuries with their location, approximate dimensions and shapes. One need not be over-fastidious in measuring all external injuries. When some specifically important marks are present on the body, however, they should be accurately measured and drawn on paper for subsequent comparison with the insulting object. A liberal use of photographic cover will help in this regard.

Skin — Note evidence of bodily reactions like hyperaemia, serum-filled bullae, etc. Record a complete description of the burnt surface. Preserve skin tissues for histopathology, ideally from burnt and adjoining un-burnt or hyperaemic areas. Note punctate marks, peppering, burns, scalds, chemical coagulation, abnormal pigmentation, frostbite and atypical lacerations at the angles of eyes and mouth. The latter are due to the wind-blast effect, especially during escape.

Mucosa — Note cherry-red colour due to exposure to carbon monoxide, sub-conjunctival haemorrhages due to negative 'g' forces, rotational changes during escape and due to whole-body linear acceleration and wind-blast effect.

Face and Eyes — Look for a flattening of features due to impact, froth in the mouth, lacerations at angles of mouth, the condition of teeth (which can help to identify the victims) and retinal haemorrhages (which can occur due to wind-blast effect and negative 'g' forces). When the body is restrained only by a torso harness, there is acute violent compression of the thorax and upper abdomen. This causes sudden displacement of blood from the right atrium and superior vena cava, with venous and capillary congestion in superficial vessels of the head and neck. In extreme cases, known as Traumatic Asphyxia, this may cause a rupture of conjunctival capillaries. This also causes "black eyes" due to deceleration against air stream in escape from aircraft. There are black eyes due to acceleration load along blood vessels of the neck, as the head is held forward.

Hands — Look for a contusion of the thenar muscles of hands, which can occur if the pilot was holding the control stick at the time of the crash. Such injuries (designated as "control injuries") to the hands and feet are useful because they indicate who was in control of the aircraft. A tight hold on the control stick at the time of the crash will cause fractures of the hand. Abrasions, contusions, soft tissue injuries and fractures occur in the area between the thumb and the index finger. There may be fractures of the metacarpals and if the impact is very severe, the proximal joint of the thumb may be crushed and the distal ulna and radius fractured. All such injuries are mostly on the inner (flexor) aspect of the hands.

Similarly, fractures in the foot may occur if the impact is transmitted through pedal controls. Thus, tarsal and metatarsal bones may be fractured, laceration of soles might occur and talar neck might be damaged (aviator's astralgus).

The following "head-to-foot" plan is suggested to avoid any inadvertent omission:

Head

1. Take special care while removing the skull cap to avoid damage that might later be mistaken for an ante-mortem injury. An electric/battery-

operated saw is very helpful in this regard.

2. Record all fractures, injuries to meninges and brain. The presence of pre-existing pathology, like cerebral aneurysms or colloid cyst of the third ventricle should be identified. The latter is often indicative of a sudden incapacitation of the pilot.
3. Explosive fractures of the skull are important. These fractures can result from intense heat during burning and are likely to be confused with traumatic fractures. However, explosive fractures of the skull involve separation of skull bones from sutures and thus can be easily differentiated from traumatic fractures.
4. Search for radiating fracture lines from foramen magnum, which occur when there is a sudden forward movement of the head (whiplash). These are easily missed unless particularly searched for.
5. In cases of intense burns, there is a splitting of the skin and separation of skull bones. In addition, cooked haematoma in the middle cranial fossa may be encountered which are usually due to post-mortem fire effects. They should be interpreted with care.
6. Immediately freeze pieces of brain tissue if hypoxia is suspected and lactic acid estimation is indicated. Lactic acid determination is only useful if brain tissue is retrieved almost immediately after the death and frozen promptly.
7. Look for the presence of ante-mortem sub-conjunctival haemorrhages, particularly in cases of attempted escape by ejection. Sub-conjunctival haemorrhages may also be encountered when intense negative 'g' is experienced.

Neck and Thorax

1. Carefully note vertebral and rib fractures with special emphasis on the fracture lines as they sometimes help to determine the direction of insulting forces. Rib fractures should be correlated with injuries to underlying organs (e.g. liver, heart and lungs) in order to differentiate between organ injuries induced by fractured ribs and those caused by deceleration forces.
2. Look for fractures of the sternum, especially at the posterior aspect, at the level of 2nd, 3rd and 4th ribs. Interestingly, if viewed from the

anterior side, the sternum can look absolutely normal. However, when the posterior surface is examined after cleaning the attached tissue, the pathologist may find a 'greenstick-like' crack. This can indicate hyperflexion of the body as a result of severe deceleration.

3. Remove the heart as a whole and open its chambers for detailed study. Look for patent foramen ovale and categorize the atherosclerotic status of coronary arteries. Search for a rupture of the heart and a laceration of the aorta, which provide very useful information. There may be laceration of the heart by crushing and stretching forces due to the impact on the precordium, especially due to forward bending. There is a 'paper bag' effect when hydrostatic forces are transmitted to the heart by way of great blood vessels, increasing the intraventricular pressure of heart to the point of rupture.[36,37] Crushing injuries of the abdomen and even lower extremities may displace blood towards the heart with sufficient force to rupture the intrapericardial portion of the aorta, lacerate valves or cause an explosive type of disruption of the wall of the left ventricle or atrium. The site of aortic lesion is usually just distal to the insertion of the obliterated ductus arteriosus and first portion of ascending aorta. Finally, ensure a proper fixation of the heart tissue for detailed histological studies. Histological findings like "focal myocarditis" are very important, as will be noted later.
4. The mechanism of the aortic injuries is very interesting. In linear acceleration/deceleration of the thorax, the central portion of the descending aorta (which is least rigidly bound) is snapped forward by the momentum of the body and mass of blood inside. There is a more rapid deceleration of the proximal part of the aorta, which is fixed by the great blood vessels of the arch and ligamentum arteriosum. Thus, great strain is exerted at its junction with the mobile descending segment. Similarly, difference in fixation and mobility of heart vis-à-vis the first portion of the ascending aorta accounts for the vulnerability of the ascending aorta at this site.[36]
5. Respiratory Tract: 80 to 85 per cent of aircraft accidents are associated with fire. Carefully dissect the larynx and tracheo-bronchial tree and

search for foreign bodies, soot or carbon particles. Note and record the condition of the lining mucosa (Kunzru & Adaval[38]). Soot particles, if found, must be carefully preserved as considerable interest is being generated in using the soot particle energy loss spectroscopic analysis to locate the site of fire and nature of burnt substance (Birky[39]). The presence of soot particles in the tracheae provides an indication that the individual was alive when exposed to fire. Their presence in the stomach further indicates swallowing action on part of the casualty and may help in ascertaining the time of survival in the smoky atmosphere.

6. Oedema of the larynx and severe inflammation of the upper respiratory passage result from inhalation of irritating and toxic fumes and, therefore, congestion and the presence of blood and froth are noteworthy.
7. Other features to note include air embolism and mediastinal emphysema, which may occur due to explosive decompression. Often corroborative evidence is sought in suspected "blast" cases. Whenever an individual is exposed to blast forces, a condition, often called "lung concussion" results, due to differential acceleration imparted to different components of lung tissue. Findings that often result from the effect of a blast are "sub-pleural haemorrhages, presenting in a definite linear pattern of rib-markings". If found, their exact location must be recorded. When these markings are present on only one side of the thorax, this finding may help in tracing the direction of blast forces to locate the place where the blast must have occurred. (Of course, other evidence to suggest a blast is the presence of burns and peppering of the skin and skin-wounds due to flying objects, which assumes greater importance when a blast is suspected.)
8. A word about preservation of lung tissue at this stage is necessary. Although pieces of all viscera should be preserved for histological examination, it is also worthwhile to preserve large portions of lung tissue for evidence of bone marrow and fat embolism. Some of these pieces will have to be examined by the "frozen section" technique. This should be kept in mind during preservation.

Abdomen

1. Note injuries to all viscera. Tear of the mesentery is very important to look for. This, along with contusion of bowel walls, gives indication of "lap-belt" injury.
2. Liver injuries must be correlated with fractured ribs. A "rupture of liver" is often recorded as due to deceleration forces when it is actually due to the jagged end of a fractured rib.
3. Examine the stomach for evidence of any pre-existing disease, like an ulcer. It is important to note the state of digestion of consumed food material. It is often prudent to preserve stomach contents for further analysis to detect the presence of any drugs.
4. Rupture of the diaphragm occurs mainly in cases of escape.

Vertebral Column and Pelvis

1. Note all fractures and dislocations for the purpose of determining the direction of forces. The exact location of injuries should be recorded and confirmed later by X-rays. An anterior wedge fracture of one or two adjacent or a series of vertebrae, usually mid-cervical or T10 to L2 area may be found in an escape from the aircraft.
2. Pelvic examination is often ignored. This can lead to the loss of valuable evidence. Dislocation of pubic symphysis may occur due to the pull of the harness. Injuries to the groin, scrotum and testes are important for further correlation with impact forces. Fractures of ischeal tuberosities are often missed. However, X-rays may reveal them if contusions and external lacerations on the buttocks are evident. Such injuries may provide information about the impact on the buttocks, which could occur for several reasons (e.g. direct impact, parachute landing).
3. If possible, collect a sample of urine. Analysis of urine for alcohol, drugs and other metabolites may be required later.

Extremities

1. Categorize all fractures noted as either open or closed. If they are bilateral, determine whether they are concomitant and point towards a particular direction of force. It is of paramount importance to note if the

fractures are haemorrhagic or bloodless. Haemorrhagic fractures denote their ante-mortem nature while bloodless fractures are usually post-mortem. If both bloodless and haemorrhagic fractures occur in the same body, it indicates that some injuries occurred when the blood circulation was intact.

2. Dislocations of shoulder and hip joints may occur due to flailing.
3. Look for contusions over the thenar muscles of the hands in aircrew victims, along with injuries to adjacent metacarpo-phalangeal joints. This is of value in determining whether the pilot was holding the control stick at the time of the crash.[40, 41]

Fractures

1. Explosive fractures of the skull are important. These fractures can be due to intense heat during burning and are likely to be confused with traumatic fractures. However, explosive fractures of the skull can cause separation of skull bones from the suture lines and can be easily distinguished from traumatic fractures.
2. Radiating fractures from the foramen magnum are seen when there is sudden forward movement of the head (whiplash). These are easily missed unless particularly looked for.
3. A typical fracture may occur on the posterior table of the sternum, indicating a sudden hyper-flexion or jack-knifing movement.
4. Vertebral fractures — There may be an anterior wedge fracture of one or two adjacent, or a series of vertebrae, usually mid-cervical or T10 to L2 area, especially in an escape from the aircraft.
5. Dislocation of shoulder or hip may result from flailing.
6. Separation of pubis symphysis is due to pull of the harness.
7. Fracture of ischeal tuberosities and ankle-bones may be observed, due to a parachute landing.
8. A fractured femur in civil airlines is often due to axial load vs. bending load: Brownson et al.[42] studied a large number of pelvic and lower limb injuries in survivors of Boeing 737-400 crashes in the UK. They highlighted that, had there been fire, these survivors might not have been able to escape. Previously, pelvic and lower limb injuries were

attributed to flailing and AXIAL LOADING at the femur. In fact, however, BENDING LOADING is the cause of femur fracture in impact aircraft accidents. In the presence of intact occupant protection systems, a femoral bending mechanism involving the front seat spar of passenger seats is a primary cause of femoral fracture in an impact aircraft accident.

9. Haemorrhagic and bloodless fractures in the same body indicate ante- and post-mortem injuries.

Fractures during such investigations are detected by gross autopsy examination as well as with radiological evidence. However, in spite of sensitive and sophisticated machines, radiography may not reveal details of fractures. In 1965, a C 123 cargo plane crashed in South Vietnam. Ten years later, osseous remains of 37 people were recovered and studied by Mann and Holland.[43] Calcanei and tali of these casualties showed variable range and pattern of perimortem fractures, which otherwise would not have been determined, had they been covered by skin and subcutaneous tissue.

CHAPTER 4

INJURY ANALYSIS AND RECURRING THEMES OF INJURY

There is nothing spectacular about the autopsy procedure and guidelines for detecting positive findings. It is a matter of "what one knows — one sees". After a great deal of experience, a pathologist gains sufficient knowledge and develops an insight into this subject. Certain recurring themes of injuries are peculiar to aviation accidents. An experienced pathologist will note these injuries and give them due importance rather than dismissing them as "insignificant" and losing vital information. A complete list of the recurring themes is difficult to compile. Many pathologists, however, make checklists of injuries and keep them handy at the time of autopsy. Some of these are summarized below:

Features of a body's outward appearance (e.g. punctate marks, burns, chemical coagulation and pigmentation) must be recorded in detail as they may be required for an evaluation of crash factors and their causes. Laceration at the angles of the mouth and eyes are characteristic of the "wind-blast effect", especially during escape. Findings in the internal organs are also critical. A contusion of the bowel wall and mesentery can indicate "lap-belt injury". Soot particles in the trachea and stomach show survival in smoke or fire (further analysis of these soot particles can give a clue to their origin and can locate the site/material that burned and its proximity to the deceased). Rib markings on the lungs suggest sudden blast effect and rupture of the diaphragm may result during escape. There are certain vulnerable spots in the heart and aorta where lacerations occur due to abrupt sudden deceleration. Explosive fracture of the skull occurs due to fire, and can be distinguished from traumatic fractures, as described in

Chapter 3. When there is sudden deceleration, the forward movement of the head (whiplash) causes typical radiating fracture hairlines from the foramen magnum. These are visible only if the bone surface is properly cleaned and closely examined. In a sudden forward "jack-knifing" movement of the body due to intense forward deceleration (especially with lap-belt in position), there is a "green stick-like" fracture on the posterior table of the sternum. This, again, has to be examined as there is no fracture on the anterior aspect of the sternum and the radiological finding is usually negative. Fractures of vertebrae and the condition of inter-vertebral discs provide useful information on the direction of the forces that have operated on the body (vertical or horizontal). A fracture of ischeal tuberosities should be observable in cases of escape. Separation of pubic symphysis occurs due to the pull of the harness. The presence of haemorrhagic and bloodless fractures in the same body may help to differentiate between injuries that were sustained when circulation was intact and those that occurred when the circulation had ceased (like those caused by terminal impact on the ground).

Ejection Injuries

To detect and assess injuries sustained during ejection from an aircraft, it is necessary for a pathologist to understand the mechanism and sequence of ejection. This mechanism and sequence of ejection is under constant improvement and sophistication.

As aircraft speed increased, manual escape became impossible and ejection as a means of escape was conceived in Sweden and developed in Germany. In the earlier systems, the pilot had to first jettison his canopy and then, a little later, pull the face-blind to eject. Upon ejection, a drogue parachute was fired to stabilise the seat and the pilot had to release his seat-restraint harness. On clearing of the seat, he had to manually deploy the parachute by pulling the 'D' ring. This process involved canopy jettisoning and further manual actions that had inherent difficulties, and the mishandling of these steps could cause injuries.

Since 1953, fully automated ejection systems have been developed wherein ejection is initiated by pulling face-blind or by a seat-pan handle.

The canopy is automatically separated, ejection and stabilisation of the seat occurs, and the seat is separated automatically at a pre-set barometric altitude with a G and time-controlled delay system automatically deploying the parachute.

These ejection systems have become very sophisticated and differ in different aircraft. To determine the possibility of incurring injuries, it is worthwhile classifying the potential hazards according to sequences involved (Barwood[44]) :

Initiation. If a face-blind is operated, it is a matter of extracting the face-blind on the front-top of the seat at top head level and pulling this down over the face. Alternatively, the process is started by pulling the seat-pan handle (positioned on the front seat pan) between the legs. During both these processes, the possibility of sustaining injury is minimal. Pilots are extensively trained in ejection drills to keep them prepared for the loads they will be experiencing. Slipping of the hand while pulling the face-blind and incorrect positioning of the elbows can result in injuries, although this has rarely occurred.

Acceleration. The dual cartridge type of gun to fire the ejection seat was developed to achieve effective tail-fin clearance. Acceptable acceleration, established using human volunteers, was 20 Gravitational acceleration applied at a rate not exceeding 200 G per second. With the increased speed of aircraft and the development of fully automated ejection systems, the system now involves a maximum of 25 G at a rate not exceeding 300 G per second with separation velocity of 80 feet per second. With the rearrangement of seat contents (the parachute being applied behind the back of the crew member and a survival pack under the seat-pan) back injuries became common due to the excessive load that was applied to the body with the spine in an adverse attitude.

The acceleration applied to the body considerably exceeds that applied to the seat. This is due to the "ejection-overshoot" provided by the compressible survival pack under the body. In addition, when the body moves downward to compress the survival pack, the tightness of the harness-restraint-straps will be reduced, resulting in loss of effective restraint. Thus, some degree of body slumping occurs in the initial stage of ejection, resulting in low-back injuries. The injury usually entails an anterior wedge fracture of one or two adjacent vertebrae or a series of vertebrae from mid-cervical to low-lumbar. The T10 to L2 area is usually more often affected. With the wedging (which is usually very minimal), displacements are rare. In earlier days, mid-thigh injuries used to occur due to pick-up of the legs by the front of the seat when the legs were pulled back off the rudder pedals and were not resting on the pack front at the time the ejection was initiated. The hard round front edge of the survival pack impacted on the back of the thigh to cause such injuries. A very narrow cockpit and damage to the outer aspect of flying boots have resulted in minor injuries to the upper and outer aspects of the knees and feet. Individual cases, involving a collision with part of the aircraft, with separated canopy, contact with the drogue system, or drogues entangled with the seat, etc. have been reported but are not "recurring themes" of injury. However, if a pathologist has to assess the "use or abuse of safety equipment" on the spot, inspection of body and safety equipment is necessary.

Airblast. Besides injuries due to hail or rain, flailing of arms may produce fracture dislocations of the upper end of the humerus, dislocation of the hip and tearing of the lateral ligaments of the knee. Other injuries due to the wind-blast effect, like conjunctival haemorrhages, have already been highlighted under recurring themes of injury. There may be superficial skin damage due to shearing forces which separate skin into layers. Friction can also produce bleeding and thermal injuries.

Free Fall. Effects of hypoxia, high wind chill and cold/frostbite can occur. Centrifugal effects due to rotation in free fall are reported and include conjunctival and retinal haemorrhages.

Separation. Impact from the separated seat and recoiling of oxygen hoses have been reported (Barwood[44]). When ejection is at a low level, the ideal stability of the seat may not be achieved and parachute extraction can take place at any attitude, producing back injury.

Parachute landing. Some fractures that result from imperfect landing have already been discussed under injuries to the vertebral column, extremities and fractures. Ekeland[45] reported a prospective study of 4,499 jumps in military parachuting. The ankle was most commonly affected and 80 per cent of injuries occurred in the lower extremities. Fourteen per cent of injured people had severe injuries such as fractures and rupture of knee ligaments. Bar-Dayan Y,[46] in a retrospective study of 43,542 military jumps, found that the overall injury rate was 0.89 per cent. The rate of major injuries was 0.21 per cent and that of minor injuries 0.68 per cent. Major injury comprised fractures, dislocations and head trauma.

Collin[47] reviewed major injuries and fatalities in USAF ejections from 1981 to 1995. Injuries have directly resulted from: (a) seat acceleration forces, (b) aerodynamic forces applied to crew members during escape through effects of wind-blast and parachute opening shock, (c) direct contact and (d) parachute landing. These injuries have usually occurred to the head, neck, cervical spine, ribs, pelvis and extremities. According to Collin, these injuries usually occur due to anomalies in ejection sequence or delayed ejection. A planned and modern seat ejection provides minimal chance for injuries.

Injuries due to Linear Deceleration

When there is a sudden deceleration with the body secured by a torso harness, an acute violent compression of the thorax and upper abdomen occurs. Consequently, there is a sudden displacement of blood from the right atrium and superior vena cava with a resultant congestion of capillaries and veins of the head or neck. (In clinical terms, this is known as "traumatic asphyxia"). This effect usually occurs in high-speed escapes from the aircraft with sudden deceleration in the ejection seat by a high-speed air stream with the head held forward. Patechial haemorrhages in the soft unsupported tissue of the face (especially peri-orbital) and conjunctiva are characteristic findings. Research on the rate of build-up, magnitude and duration of intra-thoracic and intra-abdominal pressure has shown that such transient venous pressure waves are sufficient to cause this injury.

Cardiovascular trauma entails lethal lesions of the heart and great vessels. The mechanism of such injuries is varied. There may be stabbing wounds due to ends of broken ribs, lacerations due to crushing/stretching force on impact over the precordium, impact with the instrument panel on sudden deceleration and indirect injury (e.g. contusion on the posterior wall of the heart) due to compression and consequent contact with the vertebral column. When hydrostatic forces are transmitted to the heart through great vessels, intra-ventricular pressure increases and can cause rupture. Violent compression of the abdomen or lower extremities displaces blood toward the heart with sufficient force to rupture the intra-pericardial portion of the aorta. This can lacerate valves or cause an explosive type of disruption of the walls of the left atrium or ventricle.

Sudden forceful compression of the thorax or rapid linear deceleration results in trauma to the aorta. Sites most prone to injury are just distal to the insertion of the obliterated ductus arteriosus and the first portion of the descending aorta. The central portion of the descending aorta is less rigidly fixed and during sudden linear deceleration, this part of the aorta is snapped forward by the momentum of the body and of the blood contained in the aorta. At the same time, however, the proximal aorta is fixed by the great vessels of the arch and ligamentum arteriosum. Consequently, great strain is exerted at its junction with the mobile segment to make this site vulnerable. A similar difference in "anchoring" and mobility of the heart as compared with that of the first portion of the ascending aorta makes their junction prone to injury. [36,48]

A critical analysis of these injuries is necessary not only to evaluate the trauma but also to consider the survivability vis-à-vis safety equipment provided. Lillehei[49] assessed such injuries in the victims of the Continental Flight 1713 airline disaster and suggested improvement in the passenger restraint system, based upon a study of injury patterns. Li G[50,51] also suggested a better and more effective restraint system with improved aircraft design.

Based on a large volume of data that has accumulated over a period of years, many attempts have been made to analyze the injuries sustained during fatal/non-fatal aircraft accidents. These analyses attempted to determine the pattern of injury, mechanism of causation, survivability and relationship with various factors pertaining to aircrew, passengers and aircraft. All such attempts have been directed towards prevention, which may entail improvement/modification in aircraft design, systems, life-support equipment and other protective devices.

It is interesting to note that, as early as 1964, Reals et al.[52] had reviewed the accessioned cases at the Armed Forces Institute of Pathology, Washington. These pertained to light-aircraft accidents from 1944 through 1962. Of 210 cases of such accidents with autopsies that were reviewed, 178 provided sufficient data for analysis. The average age of the pilots was found to be 34 years. Most of the light aircraft were the single-engine type. Of the 210 cases, 177 were involved in air-to-ground accidents, 2 in air-to-water, 2 in mid-air-collisions and 1 in in-flight incidence, with 28 remaining as "undetermined". In 8 cases, evidence of a pre-existing disease in the pilots was sufficient to be considered a major cause of the accident. With respect to environmental factors, hypoxia was not a cause due to low altitude but there was evidence of ante-mortem burns in a number of cases. Head injury was most common, followed by injuries to limbs. The brain was injured most often, followed in order by the aorta, liver, kidneys and heart. In some cases, the injuries might not have been fatal, but they caused incapacitation to prevent escape from the burning aircraft, finally causing death due to burning.

These authors emphasised that autopsies must be performed on all fatalities, services of a trained aviation pathologist must be requisitioned and analysis of injuries should be done in conjunction with the authorities responsible for flying safety. Similarly, at a study conducted by the Civil Aeronautics Board in the USA, coordination was recommended among pathologists, engineers, air-frame designers and safety-belt manufacturers. The study noted that most head injuries to passengers resulted from the jack-knifing motion of the body restrained by a lap-belt, causing forward movement of the head and its impact against back of the seat in front. An increase in the space between the seats, the use of shoulder harnesses and rearward facing seats were among the remedies considered.

Adaval et al.[12]conducted an analysis of the autopsies performed on air-crash fatalities over a period of 14 years at the Indian Air Force Institute of Aviation Medicine. Autopsy reports, histological/toxicological findings and reports of the Courts of Inquiry were correlated with factors such as age, aircraft type, phase of flight, the relationship of the body with the aircraft wreckage, the accident–autopsy interval, the general condition and adequacy of the body parts available, the cause and mode of death and the injury pattern. Most of the pilot casualties belonged to the age group of 21–30 years and disintegration of bodies was more likely in fighter aircraft accidents than in transport plane accidents. No disintegration was found in helicopter accidents.

There is a general impression that most fatalities occur during landing and take-off. In this study, however, only 13.4 per cent of the casualties occurred during these phases in comparison with 33 per cent due to loss of control and 43 per cent resulting from a collision with ground or water. Mason[1] also found that casualties during landing or take-off made up only 11.5 per cent. Mathur and Banerjee,[53] in their study of 200 deaths resulting from 113 fatal aircraft accidents, found that 21 per cent occurred during these phases.

Adaval et al.[12] observed that separation from or entrapment in the aircraft after the crash considerably modified the injury pattern. Entrapment may cause several types of secondary injuries, making it difficult to evaluate the trauma on primary impact and to reconstruct the sequence of events. Disintegration of bodies occurred more often when the bodies were trapped and retained in the wreckage than when they were thrown clear. Deaths due to burning, drowning and asphyxia were more frequent in the retained cases. The incidence of brain, heart and lung injuries was equal for separated and retained cases. However, injuries to the stomach, intestines, kidneys, liver and spleen were much more extensive and frequent in retained cases. Injury to the diaphragm was more common and extensive in cases of unsuccessful ejections, indicating high susceptibility of the diaphragm to deceleration trauma.

The high incidence of liver injuries in aviation accidents has been reported by many workers.[4,1] These studies found that the liver was damaged in 61 per cent of retained and 58 per cent of separated cases. The right lobe was injured more often than the left and extreme damage occurred in ejection-escape cases. Besides injury analysis, these studies also highlighted the usefulness of toxicological and histological examinations. More useful information came forth when bodies of victims were retrieved quickly and also when services of a trained aviation pathologist were requisitioned.

Whereas the studies by Adaval et al.[12] and by Mathur and Banerjee[53] were mostly restricted to Air Force aircraft accidents, Dulchavsky et al.[54] analyzed injuries following the crash of Avianca Flight 52 on Long Island, New York. They indicated multiple organ injury involving most of the organs and skeletal system in percentages and concluded that deaths were from severe head and upper body injuries, whereas unrestrained infants suffered more severe trauma. A reappraisal of current restraint and safety measures was recommended.

Li G and Baker[50] studied injury patterns of persons who died in aviation crashes in the United States in both 1980 and 1990. Fairly stable injury patterns were found at both times. Multiple injuries were the cause of death in 42 per cent of the cases, followed by head injury (22 per cent), internal injuries to the thorax, abdomen or pelvis (12 per cent), burns (12 per cent); and drowning (3 per cent). A single injury was sustained in 18 per cent of the cases, most of which were head injuries of a deceleration nature. Modifications in restraint systems and aircraft designs were suggested to make them more effective against deceleration forces.

Li G and Baker[51] tried to identify the factors associated with pilot fatalities in general aviation crashes in the USA. Over a period of 10 years in North Carolina and Maryland, 667 crashes occurred, with 276 deaths and 368 injuries. Of these, 146 (22 per cent) of the pilots-in-command died. This fatality rate was significantly higher when the crash occurred at night, away from the airport, than when it was associated with fire or when the plane was flying in instrument meteorological weather conditions. High impact forces contributed to the majority of deaths. A crashworthy fuel system and better occupant protection systems were recommended.

Needless to say, most of these analyses have been done with the objective of assessing the mechanism of injuries, sequencing the events, understanding the survivability of the insult vis-à-vis aircraft design, structural failure and safety equipment available.[55] Important suggestions to improve the design and to provide better and safer restraint systems have been made with the active involvement of aviation pathologists in the multi-linear approach.

In India, one civil airliner crashed into the sea almost immediately after take-off. Bodies of passengers were recovered within the next two days. While conducting autopsies on these fatalities, the author found a distinct pattern. The bodies were all transected from waist level. Faces and heads were badly mutilated and flattened. X-rays of the thorax also showed that spines were transected at the level of the lap-belt but inter-vertebral spaces were intact. There was no telescoping of the vertebrae. These findings indicated that there was sudden forward deceleration at the time when all passengers were sitting with their lap-belts fastened. Consequently, there was sudden forward movement of heads, which banged against the rear of the seats in front, while transection of the bodies occurred due to fastened seat belts. X-rays also showed intact inter-vertebral spaces as the impact was in the antero-posterior direction. Further investigations showed that the aircraft nosedived and crashed on the sea surface due to a technical fault.

Figure 4.1 below shows a typical finding, as stated above, wherein the head is more or less smashed and the body is transected at waist level.

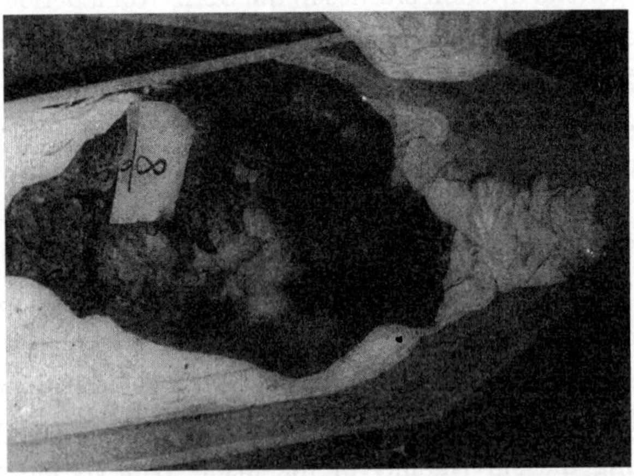

Figure 4.1: A body transected at waist with missing head

Similarly, an X-ray of the spine showed more or less intact inter-vertebral spaces but a transection at waist level, as shown in Figure 4.2 .

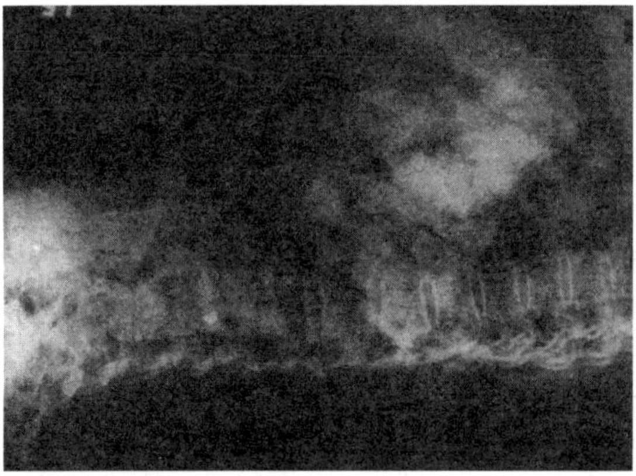

Figure 4.2: X-ray spine showing no significant telescoping of vertebrae

Assessment of Burns

Most aircraft accidents are associated with fire. Although in a large majority of cases, fire is a post-crash complication, some accidents are caused by in-flight fire. Fire attains severe intensity due to the presence of highly inflammable material. Burns sustained by the occupants are frequently to be assessed by the pathologists, primarily to differentiate between ante-mortem and post-mortem burns. When there is intact circulation and respiration while sustaining burns, there are bound to be some vital reactions in the body, which can be seen during the autopsies.[38] If the aircraft crashes on the ground and catches fire, there is usually instantaneous death of the occupants and thus there is no time for the tissue reactions to develop. Unfortunately, many bodies incinerated after death have been classified erroneously as having died from burning, due to inadequate examination and non-availability of an expert pathologist. On the other hand, Salomone[56] reports that while investigating the Galaxy Flight 203 crash site near Reno, Nevada, and correlating autopsy and toxicological findings, 68 persons died at the scene and of these, the majority had survived the impact but succumbed to toxic gas and fire.

A thorough autopsy along with histological and toxicological examinations is stressed by many workers to bring out useful information in problematic cases.[1] Modi[57] lists lines of redness, vesication and reparative processes as evidence of burns sustained during life. According to him, redness occurs "immediately" after burns and vesication forms within an hour. Anderson[58] emphasizes that the earliest cytological evidence of hyper-thermal injury is a redistribution of the fluid and solid components of nuclei followed by nuclear swelling due to imbibing of fluid, rupture of nuclear membranes and pyknosis. Cytoplasm of the cells becomes first granular and later homogeneously coagulated. Collagen loses its fibrillar character and is seen as a dense homogeneous gel. Thermally denatured cells have a low pH and thus a greater affinity to basic stains.

Although many forensic pathologists are confronted with the problem of differentiating ante-mortem from post-mortem burns, the situation is somewhat different in aircraft accident investigations. If the aircrew are subjected to in-flight fire and incapacitated, the aircraft is likely to crash within a few seconds. This interval of a few seconds is important in this type of investigation. So far, there appears to be no established method of differentiating between the ante-mortem and post-mortem nature of burns when the duration between exposure to burns and death is only a few seconds. Adaval et al.[59] have assessed findings in 305 autopsies in which burns/incineration were found in 125 cases. However, due to inadequate investigations and non-utilisation of a trained aviation pathologist, ante-mortem burns could be confirmed with certainty in only 6 of 11 cases.

Mason[1] has applied certain criteria which should be taken into account for overall assessment, such as froth from the nose and mouth, macroscopic venous congestion, carbon particles in the trachea and stomach, microscopic congestion of blood vessels, cerebral vessel congestion, pulmonary histology, skin histology and carboxyhaemoglobin estimation in the blood and tissue. Widespread and obvious venous congestion is universal, and its absence might cast considerable doubt on the diagnosis of ante-mortem burns. The absence of carbon particles in the trachea, lungs or stomach does not preclude a diagnosis of death from burning as a high-intensity flash fire might not leave such evidence. Microscopic congestion of organs is also a universal finding, which is more marked in the spleen and brain. However, similar findings are also encountered in other forms of asphyxial deaths and cerebral deceleration trauma. This finding should, therefore, be interpreted with due caution. In the lungs, intra-alveolar oedema with moderate exudation of phagocytes is described. Carbon pigment can sometimes be seen mixed with blood and has to be especially investigated. Histological findings of the skin are very important from a diagnostic point of view but may be obscured by charring and other artifacts associated with burning. Anderson[58] emphasises that the earliest evidence of hyper-thermal injury is functional rather than structural. Besides vascular congestion, mild infiltration with inflammatory cells may be found. If there is exposure to intense heat, however, the superficial area could become so rapidly fixed in a state of contraction that such changes might not be seen. Thus, a pathologist might have to look for them at a deeper level. Anyway, due to its variability (e.g. regression after death) hyperemia makes it a doubtful marker of ante-mortem burns. Many workers have emphasised the value of blood or tissue carboxy-haemoglobin levels in assessing deaths due to burning (Blackmore[60]). Glantz et al.[61] recommended a 10 per cent level as a criterion but the absence of such levels does not preclude the possibility of ante-mortem burns. On the other hand, false positive results may be obtained as a result of contamination of the cockpit air with carbon monoxide, with consequent incapacitation and post-crash fire.

Analysis of soot particles recovered from the trachea, lungs and stomach has become vital, as electron energy-loss spectroscopic analysis of these particles gives us valuable information on the origin and nature of fire (Mitchelson,[62] Chaturvedi[63]). These studies are referred to in the chapter on toxicology of carbon monoxide.

In most crashes, victims die as a result of impact injuries well before they sustain burns. Merely finding soot in the mouth/nose and oropharynx does not necessarily mean that the individual was alive when exposed to fire, as this can be due to agonal respiratory excursion. However, soot in the distal trachea (below the vocal cords) and bronchi does suggest ante-mortem exposure to fire. The pathologist is advised to study multiple sections (gross and microscopic) to ascertain this. He should also remember that even when a live individual is exposed to fire, there may be, in some instances, a laryngeal spasm. This prevents soot from entering the respiratory tract. In such cases, even carboxyhaemoglobin (COHb) levels may not be high. The picture below (Figure 4.3) shows distinct soot particles in the larynx and trachea in a case of in-flight fire. This was corroborated by the findings of intensely congested blood vessels seen in the histological sections (Figure 4.4).

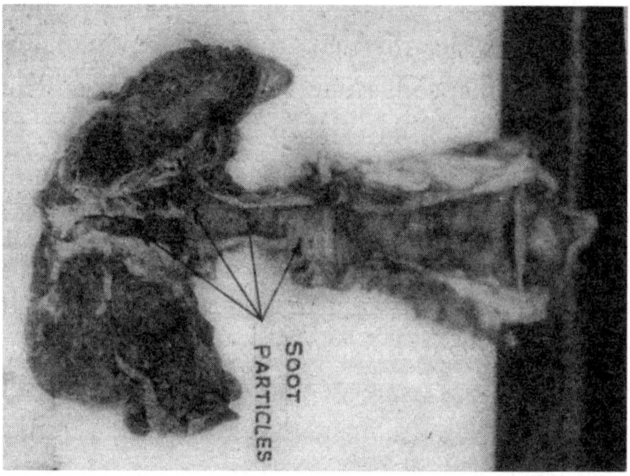

Figure 4.3: Dissected trachea showing soot particles

A histological section from the same case shows intense congestion of blood vessels in the trachea and larynx (Figure 4.4)

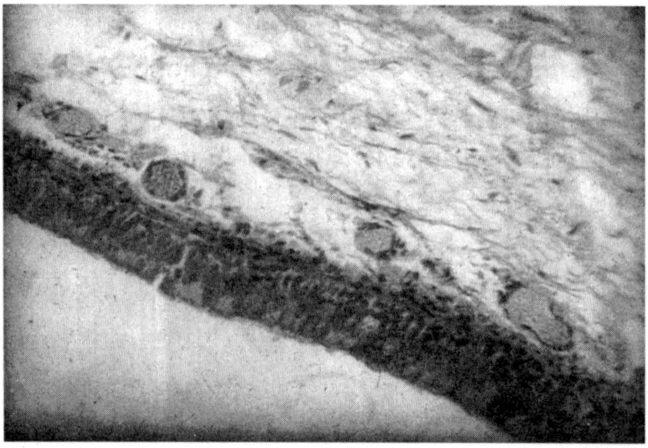

Figure 4.4: Histological section of trachea showing congested blood vessels

When associating COHb levels with thermal injuries, it might be noted that up to 6 per cent blood levels can be found in chronic smokers and about 7 per cent in people living in industrial areas. Thus, levels above 10 per cent should be regarded as significant. These levels depend upon the duration of exposure to fire and space enclosing the fire and victim. Levels from 30 per cent to 60 per cent are encountered in transport aircraft and from 10 per cent to 30 per cent in smaller aircraft. According to Dunne and Meekin,[64] a level of 30 per cent can generally be seen in survival of 1 to 17 minutes.

Some changes in the charred bodies due to intense heat can mislead a pathologist. There may be heat-induced fractures of bones of extremities, explosive fractures of the skull and "cooked haematoma" in the epidural space. Due to dominant contractions of the flexor muscles, the body may assume a "pugilistic" attitude, which can be misleading.

Drowning

When a fatal accident occurs on the water surface, the pathologist is often asked to determine whether death was due to injuries or as a result of drowning. In such cases, the investigator should find out whether the deceased knew how to swim. If traumatic injuries are minor and non-disabling, the verdict may be in favour of drowning. In borderline cases, detailed investigations may be necessary, as suggested by Thompson.[65] A mushroom of froth on the nose/mouth, petechial haemorrhages in conjunctiva, wrinkled skin of hands and feet, congested lungs due to aspirated water and petechial sub-pleural haemorrhages are common findings. Death due to drowning should be decided only after a careful assessment of all positive and negative findings and the exclusion of other causes, as very few features are diagnostic of death by drowning. Alteration in the blood volume and blood electrolyte contents is one factor that has been suggested in this context.

The study of "diatoms" deserves special mention as this may give vital information in cases of suspected death due to drowning. Conventionally, drowning is established when the lungs are found to contain water in which an individual drowns. In aviation fatalities, due to severe trauma, the chest cavity may be opened to allow direct access of water in the lungs, rendering it difficult to establish drowning. When death is due to drowning, water is inhaled and through damaged capillaries in the alveoli, some of this water enters blood circulation. Consequently, certain sand particles and algae circulate in the blood and get deposited in the end of long bones like the femur, where they can be detected by phase contrast microscopy. Diatoms, which are tiny one-celled chlorophyll-bearing plants in the sea's plankton, especially in cold waters of big rivers and seas, are seen by techniques that involve the digestion of a portion of tissue with acid followed by examination of sediment under the microscope. They can also be seen in routine histological sections stained by the Hematoxylin and Eosin technique. Particles of sand provide useful information. These require phase contrast microscopy to detect the configuration of a sand particle as recovered from the body and to compare it with the structure of sand particles recovered from the water bed. Collection of water from the sea-bed may be necessary to study the type of diatoms present there. Sometimes after drowning, however, the body may drift to some other area of the water and diatoms may not conform to those found in the body. This must be established by circumstantial evidence. Preservation of ends of long bones for detecting diatoms is undertaken only when drowning is suspected, and not as a routine.

CHAPTER 5

INVESTIGATION OF AIRLINE DISASTERS IN INDIA AND ABROAD

System of Investigation

There is a very comprehensive and efficient system for investigating fatal aircraft accidents in the Armed Forces of India. Investigations are conducted under the Ministry of Defence and specific services, such as the Air Force, Navy or Army. A Court of Inquiry is constituted, in which specialists from flying, technical and other concerned branches are nominated as members. A medical officer, who is a specialist in aviation medicine is also a member. A service pathologist who conducts autopsies and histopathological and toxicological investigations is not a member of the Court of Inquiry and this gives him/her freedom to work independently. The specialist in aviation medicine acts as a coordinating agency between the pathologist and the Court. This is quite similar to the procedure adopted by the RAF in the UK.

The set-up for civil aircraft accident investigation is different, however. As air travel is becoming a more and more common mode of transportation, safety levels are being stepped up. Fatalities per 100 million passenger-kilometres are declining. However, with further increase in civil airline traffic and the introduction of larger aircraft, one must be cautious in evaluating these statistics. Rates can be calculated for fatal accidents, the total number of fatalities vis-à-vis miles flown, hours during which the aircraft was airborne and the number of passengers travelling. Although accident rates may be falling, the number of fatalities may gradually be mounting due to increased aviation activity and increased mileage flown. Figures may vary, but there is no doubt that a substantial percentage of direct or indirect causes of these accidents is due to the "human factor". Time and again, a medical investigation, particularly using a pathologist's approach, has contributed significantly to flight safety. Sometimes, a lead to the cause of accident has been provided, confirming evidence deduced from other disciplines. At other times, negative evidence has excluded a suspected human factor.

Most civil aircraft accidents involve a mass disaster. With larger aircraft, the fatality figures in a single accident are on the increase and, therefore, a detailed examination of human remains is very important. When flights are international, other factors arise. For example, the persons involved may be of several nationalities, the accident may occur outside the victim's home countries, the machine may be owned and operated by a country other than the one in which the accident occurs, and investigative facilities at the accident site may be difficult to access.

Stevens[2] recommended a pre-planned and organised effort in such situations that would involve:

(a) The International Civil Aviation Organization
(b) The commission appointed to inquire into the accident, in the state in which the accident occurred.
(c) The local legal authority under whose jurisdiction the accident occurred.
(d) Local police and rescue organisations.
(e) Local doctors or pathologists appointed for investigation, autopsies, etc.
(f) The airline whose aircraft was involved.
(g) Relatives of the deceased.

When the airlines involved are from India, the investigative machinery and process is channelled through the Director General of Civil Aviation (DGCA) and is governed by Indian laws. The role of the International Civil Aviation Organization (ICAO), however, should be mentioned. Article 26 of the Chicago Convention indicates that,

> "in the event of an accident to an aircraft of a contracting state and involving death/serious injury/serious technical defect in aircraft or navigational facilities, the state in which accident occurs will institute an inquiry into the circumstances of the accident; in accordance, so far as its laws permit, with the procedure which may be recommended by ICAO. The state in which the aircraft is registered shall

> be given opportunity to appoint the observers to be present at the inquiry and the state holding the inquiry shall report the findings to that state."

Under this Article, therefore, the state in which the aircraft is registered is given the opportunity to appoint observers to be present at the inquiry. Annexure B, passed in 1966, permits such observers only to visit the scene of accident, examine the wreckage, interrogate the witnesses and peruse the documents. There is no mention of the role of medical doctors and pathologists as accredited advisors or the extent of their involvement. Similarly, the *Manual of Aircraft Accident Investigation*, published by ICAO, devotes the greater part to general points and examination of wreckage. Although the value of medical evidence is highlighted, the emphasis on "autopsy" is quite mild. This does not conform to the basic principle of medical investigation. This is especially true in light of the fact that in many countries, investigation is labelled as "incomplete" if an autopsy is not performed.

Under Standing Orders of the British Government, in all fatal aircraft accidents, civil or military, the Department of Aviation Pathology at the Institute of Pathology & Tropical Medicine, RAF, Halton (UK) is invariably involved. An aviation pathologist goes to the scene of every accident being investigated, either personally carries out the autopsies or observes the autopsies being carried out by the Coroner's pathologist, makes detailed notes on the autopsy findings, takes photographs of bodies/wreckage, collects specimens for toxicological and histopathological investigations, and finally, having considered all aspects of the accident in consultation with Board of Inquiry, submits a report either to the Board of Trade itself or to the Ministry of Defence, as the case may be.

Realising the importance of a "multi-linear approach" and group system of investigation, the US National Transport Safety Board has streamlined this procedure by earmarking the participating parties and institutions. In addition to operational, weather, air traffic control and witness groups, a "human factor" group is responsible for the aero-medical and crash injury aspects of the investigation. The Federal Aviation Administration (FAA) has developed a nationwide plan under which on-site investigations by pathologists and autopsy facilities are mandatory. In the UK, the Accident Investigation Branch (AIB) laid down a similar group system. The official international definition of this system indicates that its primary purpose is to establish the facts pertinent to an accident by making use of the specialised knowledge of the participating individuals and to ensure that any given aspect is neither unduly emphasised nor neglected.

To summarize:

(a) If the crash occurred in a country that is an ICAO member, investigations on the lines recommended by *Manual of Aircraft Accident Investigation* of ICAO would be conducted, and are the responsibility of the host country.

(b) If the host country is not a member of ICAO, then the modalities must be worked out by negotiations.

(c) The country of registration may send an accredited representative as observer or additional advisors as required (e.g. a pathologist, a Senior Inspector of the Accident Investigation Board from the Ministry of Aviation). These visiting investigators have a clearly defined status.

In the United States of America, airline accident investigations are conducted solely by the Civil Aeronautics Board (CAB) and Accident Investigating Branch of Board of Trade (AIB), using a team of invited specialists. In major accidents, the Board appoints a Chief Inspector-in-charge and assigns certain specialists to the investigation from various fields such as power plant structures, human factors, maintenance, operations, meteorology, systems and witnesses. These individuals are assigned to various groups headed by CAB specialists. Each group works independently and then coordinates with the others.

The human factors group is headed by a CAB investigator and has representatives from the Armed Forces Institute of Pathology (AFIP) Washington DC, Federal Aviation Agency (FAA), Aircraft Carrier and Airline Pilots' Associations and Air Frame Manufacturers. It is responsible for determining all medical facts, conduction of autopsies, liaison with the coroner for autopsies and rendering help for the same. It also considers the possibility of sudden incapacitation of the air crew due to medical or toxic factors. This human group also considers survivability, prevention of injuries, location of fatalities, identification, seating documents, seat-safety belt failure, structural damage vis-à-vis injuries, etc. Identification of casualties is conventionally done by clothing, documents, jewellery, medical findings, visual appearance, dental records etc.

Many accidents occur due to human failure rather than technical reasons. This failure is usually due to an error or omission by the pilot or aircrew. However, they are often not at fault, as the failure could result from inherent limitations of human response, adversities due to the atmospheric environment, or health limitations.

Preparedness, Teamwork and Liaison

In the US Air Force, an aerospace pathologist on call is notified as soon as possible following a fatal air crash. Such pathologists are always on call at OAFME. They coordinate with their civil counterparts and provide them with necessary help.

An ongoing state of preparedness for air-crash investigation is vital. Higher civil or military aviation authorities should draw up an accident investigation plan well in advance and sort out all inherent legal and administrative bottlenecks. Areas of jurisdiction of military and civil authorities should be clearly marked, as most fatal crashes fall under civil jurisdiction. Such issues should also be discussed with local authorities well in advance. Medical investigation procedures and the roles of the local civil medical officer, military doctor and aviation pathologist, should be specified in writing so that last-minute legal technicalities do not get in the way of a smooth conduction of the investigation.

Before the aviation pathologist reaches the accident scene, the role of the local medical officer (flight surgeon/squadron medical officer/state medical officer/doctor designated by civilian medical authorities) is of paramount importance. This officer may be the first doctor to reach the site of accident. Besides providing first aid to the injured and facilitating their evacuation to the hospital, the doctor should exercise the utmost care to preserve valuable evidence. In this respect, the local medical officer's role is complementary to that of the pathologist. Using liberal photographic cover, this person should ensure that vital evidence is not disturbed. Positions of the bodies at the crash site, their relation with aircraft parts/debris and the state of flying clothing are among the pieces of photographically recordable evidence that might come in handy for the pathologist later on.

When an accident occurs within a military jurisdiction, concerned defence authorities can authorise autopsies. However, there may be partial jurisdiction (e.g. aircraft from armed forces crashing in a civilian area) when close coordination of concerned authorities is necessary. In the case of pure civilian jurisdiction, local district/police/judicial officers may authorise autopsies. Many times, civil authorities insist that they will conduct the autopsies (even though they may not have a pathologist, let alone an aviation pathologist!). In such cases, an aviation pathologist from Defence may be inducted as an observer and his expertise utilised. In India, the Director General of Civil Aviation (DGCA) may help to involve a trained aviation pathologist in the investigation.

It is emphasised again that to do justice to his work, the aviation pathologist must have access to the information on man, machine and mission. As autopsy is not an isolated investigation; authentic and to-the-point information on the pilot's case history (which should include his personal habits, activities on the previous day including the type of meal taken, possibility of alcohol intake, prolonged duty hours if any, family/ medical history, interpersonal relationships, occupational stress etc.), information on the last flight, flight-path and manoeuvres which could cause sudden incapacitation would be helpful in the final analysis. Physical, physiological and psychological factors and their role in aircrew–aircraft balance, must be understood in order to gain insight into the causation of accidents that are often labelled as due to "pilot error" or "undetermined cause". The entire gamut of information may not be available to the pathologist immediately. However, some vital information pertinent to the accident may be provided quickly, with other facets made available by the time of the final analysis.

A pathologist's experience in such investigations is of paramount importance. A problem can lie with the organisation, which can create legal and administrative bottlenecks that prevent full utilisation of this discipline. Most developed countries are now insisting on the inclusion of an aviation pathologist in their team. To highlight the necessity of a multi-linear approach, a schematic depiction of facets, emphasised by Mason,[1] is illustrated in Table 5.1.

Table 5.1: Correlation of findings of medical investigations with other disciplines

	⟷	
Medical History Conditions that could produce sudden incapacitation **Autopsy, Radiological & Toxicological Cover** Rule out organic disease Detect recurring themes of injuries **Histopathology & Toxicology** Rule out organic diseases Detect possible medical causes which could cause sudden incapacitation Sequence the injuries, differentiate between ante and post-mortem injuries such as burns Ascertain survival time after injury	⟷	**Environmental Factors** Environmental factors (around the aircrew and passengers) **Structural damage to aircraft** Correlation with findings of engineers and other system specialists **Use/abuse of safety equipment** Life-support system failure Rescue Facilities Correlate with promptness of rescue operations

The foregoing scheme is deduced from Mason's definition of Aviation Accident Pathology as the "comprehensive study of aviation fatalities whereby the medical history of the casualty and the findings at autopsy can be correlated with the environmental factors, the structural or other damage to the aircraft and the use or abuse of equipment, so that a complete picture of the accident may be formed".

To quote some examples: If a pathologist finds high levels of carboxyhaemoglobin in the blood of a fatality, there may be associated evidence of an in-flight fire or leak of exhaust fumes in the cockpit/passenger compartment. Similarly, if there is evidence of hypoxia on toxicological grounds, the oxygen system of the aircraft may be checked. Serious ejection/parachute injuries can be associated with use/abuse of safety equipment (injuries characteristic of sudden decompression may be correlated with structural damage to the aircraft). Sometimes, there is no evidence of any technical failure and the cause of death remains uncertain. Such incidents are often attributed to "pilot error" or "human failure". Under such circumstances, it is advisable to check the medical history of the pilot and rule out the possible medical causes for sudden incapacitation. Thus, the interaction of the pathologists with other investigating non-medical groups is vital, as they can contribute by:

(a) Identifying natural diseases or abnormalities that could cause relative incapacitation of operating crew, to highlight a possible or probable medical cause.
(b) Identifying a "probable" non-medical cause of accident, if found.
(c) Obtaining medical evidence to suggest events that could have occurred in aircraft before accident (e.g. ante-mortem burns, fat and bone marrow embolism)
(d) Identifying the sequence of events surrounding the accident (e.g. when the aircraft was airborne, when it impacted on ground or water).
(e) Establishing the medical survivability of casualties.

Many reports highlight the role of a pathologist and the benefits of a multi-linear approach. Gregersen et al.[66] reported such an instance when the crash of the Partnair 340/580 in the Skagerrak was investigated. Medical evidence showed that the aircraft, with 55 people on board, crashed into the sea without any warning. Medical investigation was aimed at identification of all 55 fatalities and also the cause of accident. Of these fatalities, 31 were immediately recovered from the sea and 19 were recovered from the sea or shore after about a month. Injuries in the two groups differed and indicated that the aircraft had broken up in mid-air. Thus, the first group dropped into the sea after a free fall and the other remained in the wreckage. There was no evidence on the bodies to suggest fire or explosion. It was later found that the aircraft had broken up due to a structural failure in the tail section. These investigations remind us of the famous Comet disaster investigation reported by Armstrong et al.[6]

White et al.[67] reported the effects of structural failure on injuries sustained in an M1 Boeing 737 disaster. Out of 126 occupants, 10 escaped uninjured while 116 sustained injuries ranging from simple bruising to fatal crushing trauma. The degree of injury and likelihood of death was proportional to the local structural damage in the aircraft. Severe limb injuries were seen in the forward section of the wreckage where the floor had failed. Many severe head injuries were thought to be due to falling overhead lockers and unrestrained cabin furniture. Consequently, valuable information was brought forth to help plan the future prevention of such injuries. McMeekin[55,68] has also reported patterns of injury in fatal aircraft accidents.

Disaster Plan and Pathologist

To utilise the services of medical personnel in air disasters, "disaster plans" and drills are of immense help. Although these drills are nothing but rehearsals, they give us an insight into our competence and limitations. The following factors relevant to such a drill should be provided:

(a) A proper disaster plan ready under an appropriate chain of command. This plan should be properly coordinated with the police so that the work of the pathologist is facilitated. This should also enable the coroner to provide proper autopsy and allied facilities.
(b) Pre-training of all involved personnel.
(c) Adequate lay-out facilities.
(d) Mortuary, autopsy and refrigeration facilities.

(e) The establishment of a secretariat to help the pathologist record observations made at the accident site, e.g. clothing, personal possessions, dental charting and autopsy findings. This secretariat should also record other information, like physical characteristics, dental records, clothing, jewellery and description from relatives of the deceased, flight manifest and seat assignment.

Lacunae in the System

The aforementioned system is prevalent in many developed countries and is totally streamlined (McCarty[69]). In many developing countries, however, the situation is far from satisfactory. The lacunae in the system that can considerably limit the pathologist's work include the following:

(a) The pathologist is rarely able to go to the scene of accident immediately after the accident. This is in contrast with the mobility of "go teams" in countries that reach the site of accident within a couple of hours. This fact has been highlighted for quite some time (Stevens[2,70,71]). Even in many developed countries, where special aircraft are readily available to reach the site of the accident, the pathologist is taken there only after considerable delay. This is unacceptable.

(b) Situational factors such as the relation of bodies to the aircraft or the condition of the wreckage are often not known to the pathologist, as the bodies have already been removed and the wreckage has been handled by others by the time he or she arrives. This does not allow the pathologist to evaluate injuries in the context of structural components, fire, aircraft parts and toxic factors that could have operated.

(c) When an accident occurs, any pathologist available is hastily sent to conduct the investigation. Such a pathologist may not have been trained in Aviation Accident Pathology and thus may not be able to do full justice to the task. Cullen[72] cites Annexure 13 of the Convention on International Civil Aviation, which recommends that the autopsies be conducted by aviation pathologists and that they should not only aim at identification of casualties. That is, reconstruction of the accident, injury analysis, evaluation of safety equipment and medico-legal aspects must also be thoroughly covered. This can be achieved only if the services of a trained pathologist are utilised.

(d) Data available to the pathologist is often inadequate, making it impossible to correlate with other factors.

(e) On-the-spot autopsy equipment is not available and toxicological support, like facilities to collect samples and refrigeration/ice-boxes, etc. is inadequate.

Remedial Measures

To remedy the aforementioned problems, the following steps should be taken:

(a) The pathologist should be able to reach the site of accident immediately.

(b) Full relevant circumstances of the accident should be made available to the pathologist.

(c) A portable autopsy kit should accompany the pathologist for an "on-the-spot" autopsy.

(d) Adequate facilities for collection of samples, storage at required temperature and expeditious transportation to assigned laboratories must be available.

(e) For such facilities, a system must evolve, preferably by establishing Regional Aviation Pathology Cells, from where such facilities may be availed.

Kunzru et al.[25] suggested a comprehensive set-up under such situations. They recommended that all fatal air crashes (civil or military) should be investigated by a team of specialists. A specialist in aviation medicine, assisted by a local medical officer, should be part of this team. Autopsies are a must and should be conducted by experienced aviation pathologists with close liaison between the medical officer and medical members of courts of inquiry, who will be able to provide necessary information on the crash situation. Clear instructions and authority for the movements of each member should exist and the status of each member of the team, vis-à-vis total investigations, should be clearly defined.

Identification of Fatalities and the Pathologist

It is surprising that the necessity of identification is not fully appreciated after a fatal air crash, especially when bodies are mutilated. Body parts are often labelled as not-identifiable and are disposed of in various containers or coffins. Identification is necessary for personal, sentimental, social and legal reasons and authorities have often been assigned the task of identification. This is, therefore, not a primary duty of the pathologist. Nevertheless, it is sometimes necessary for a pathologist to become involved in this for reasons mentioned below.

It is necessary to identify the bodies of pilots and other aircrew in order to detect the evidence of pre-existing disease and to ascertain any cause of sudden incapacitation. In passenger aircraft accidents, identification of fatalities helps to assign them to their respective seats. Injuries/burns sustained by passengers who were seated in a particular part of the passenger compartment will provide clues to structural failure, fire and even explosion. In flight, if an emergency is pre-heralded, airhostesses and stewards are found to be sitting in their assigned seats with lap-belts secured. However, if there is a sudden catastrophe, their bodies will be found unsecured. Thus, the identification of these individuals is also necessary. Finally, when a blast with explosives is suspected, the bodies of some passengers sitting nearby will have peppering of the skin and shrapnel injuries. The seating plan will indicate where such passengers were sitting, making it easier to look for incriminating evidence.

For these reasons, it is necessary for a pathologist to be involved in the process of identification. Stevens[71] feels that the pathologist may either be in charge of the identification team or appointed as one of its members. In military air crashes, identification does not pose as great a problem, as the particulars of flyers are known and bodies bear uniform or rank insignia. More problems are encountered in passenger airline crashes, especially when bodies are grossly mutilated.

There are many simple as well as sophisticated methods of identification and these are to be used when required. First, bodies can sometimes be identified by visual means, i.e. recognition of facial and other features by relatives/people known to the deceased. This may not always be possible because of disfigurement or mutilation. Even in the absence of gross injuries, sometimes bodies present a distorted appearance due to exposure to sun and vagaries of weather. Thus, visual identification is useful only in cases where the appearance of bodies is reasonably well preserved.

One of the most important clues is obtained by personal effects of the fatalities. It is unfortunate that when bodies are brought for investigations/autopsies, clothing is removed and dumped on one side without attaching identification tags. This makes it difficult to assign a particular item to the corresponding body. In my personal experience, I have seen such lapses committed by poorly educated paramedical staff. Garments/dresses, even if found scanty, provide valuable clues, like name-tags, tailor's labels, dry-cleaner's marks and specific designs of aircrew dress. Similarly, items of jewellery may have inscriptions and even a small fragment of paper may be useful in establishing identity.

Before conducting the autopsy, the pathologist makes a note of personal details of the casualty viz. colour of skin/eyes, identification marks like moles, and also evidence of post-surgical effects/pre-existing diseases, which may come handy in identification. Dental identification is a very important aspect and should be closely followed. Teeth that are present, extracted, missing or with restoration treatment can be compared with available dental information on record. However, in developing countries, such records are seldom maintained. Even in cases of pilots belonging to the Armed Forces, updated dental records are sometimes not available. In addition to dental X-rays, radiographic evidence of old fractures, surgical procedures on bones and presence of any other pathology can sometimes be helpful. The need to subject all bones to X-rays and to maintain records was indicated in our previous discussion of autopsy procedures. In the case of children, these records may also be useful for establishing age.

In earlier days, the fingerprinting of fatalities was not recommended as fingerprint records were not routinely maintained for all citizens. At present, however, there should be no hesitation in recommending this procedure for all casualties. Serology and DNA studies are undertaken only in exceptional circumstances and therefore, are not recommended as a routine procedure. Noting all these findings and keeping an accurate record is obviously laborious, and so the pathologist must develop his own methodology and seek assistance from staff. It would be worthwhile to make a room adjacent to the autopsy room available, where all findings can be compiled and placed on record. Computer software could also be designed for this purpose.

CHAPTER 6

INVESTIGATION IN CASES OF BIRDSTRIKE

Birdstrike to a flying aircraft is a common but serious hazard. Air crashes and deaths due to bird hits have been known to occur since the early days of aviation and are still one of the most serious problems for flight safety. In the Indian Air Force, major accidents and incidents have been attributed to birdstrikes, resulting in the loss of both lives and aircraft. Between 1975 and 1986, 431 incidents of birdstrike were reported, with consequent damage to aircraft in 409 cases and loss of aircraft in 34 cases (Vidyasagar[73]). Damage occurred mostly to air-intake and engine-inlet areas followed by the nose-cone, the leading edge of the wing and the wind shield. The aircraft involved were mostly MiG and Jaguars. Birdstrikes were more frequent during the circuit and low-level, high-speed flying normally carried out by fighter or attack aircraft. In the US Air Force alone, more than 2,000 birdstrikes were reported in one year (Defusco[74]). The overall birdstrike rate was 69.9 per 100,000 flying hours. Air Force cargo and fighter or attack aircraft were again involved more frequently. Cargo aircraft were also affected due to their low-level flying. Wind-shield/canopy strikes were most frequent, followed by engine, nose and wings. Half of such incidents occurred in the airfield environment and almost all occurred at an altitude below 3,000 feet.

In non-fatal incidents when aircraft lands safely, the pilot provides an eyewitness account of the bird hit, damage to the aircraft is actually seen and there is supportive evidence such as bird feathers. Consequently, no further investigations are needed. When the accident is fatal, however, the aircraft is often abandoned and no other supportive evidence is available, except for the presence of blood on the aircraft. It then becomes necessary to establish whether this blood is of avian or human origin. The ambiguity arises most often when there is evidence of blood on the windshield but there are associated injuries to occupants as well. It is my experience that in such cases, a scraping of dried blood is brought to the pathologist with a request to determine whether it is avian or human. The collection of such samples is often not proper. That is, there is considerable delay in the collection of samples that are invariably contaminated and subject to vagaries of weather and heat due to associated fire. Thus, the identification of avian blood/tissue assumes great importance in selected cases and, therefore, a pathologist should be well versed with the procedures involved. Various methods to identify avian blood were assessed by Mathur and Adaval[75] and are worth summarizing.

Naked eye examination

Finding blood-coloured stains or liquid should not lead to the assumption that it is blood, as many substances can give an erroneous impression of blood. Brownish discoloration of the windshield and cracks with feathered edges are often erroneously taken as tell-tale signs of a bird hit.[76] Aviation fuel/oils mixed with soil and impressions produced by the bark of a tree can impart a brownish colour, resembling blood stains. It is, therefore, necessary to make use of more objective and specific methods.

Microscopic Examination

This is applicable only if the sample is fresh, as the test is based upon the appearance of red blood cells peculiar to avian blood (usually nucleated RBC). Scrapings from the suspected material are placed on a microscope-glass slide and a drop or two of distilled water is added. After allowing a period of 5 minutes for the cells to imbibe water and enlarge in size, a drop of 1 per cent methylene blue in water is added and mixed. A cover slip is applied and after 5 minutes the cells are examined under the microscope. Nucleated cells will appear as elliptical/oval cells with blue cytoplasm and a dark round nucleus. If the preparation is unstained, only elliptical/ovoid cells are seen with a faint "ghost" nucleus in an occasional cell.

Chemical Tests

Most laboratories use the Benzidine Test to detect blood. This is based on the ability of peroxidase present in the "haeme" moiety of haemoglobin to catalyze decomposition of organic peroxides. These, in turn, oxidise the reagent to produce a blue colour. This test is very sensitive and can detect haemoglobin in concentrations as low as 2 or 3 ppm. The disadvantage is that the test is not specific and false-positive results occur with many animal proteins (bone, brain, saliva, mucous etc.), products of plants (apples, beans, asparagus, potatoes, radish, turnip etc.) and chemicals like rust, soil, copper sulphate, potassium-dichromate and some bleaches. Thus, if this test is performed on the suspected sample and turns out to be negative, the presence of blood (avian or otherwise) is virtually ruled out. However, a positive test does not mean that blood is present. Most of the samples received from air-crash sites are soiled and contaminated. Consequently, the usefulness of this test is limited.

Haemochromogen Crystal Test

This test is more specific for blood. The Takayama reagent is prepared by mixing 3 ml each of 10 per cent sodium hydroxide, pyridine and saturated solution of glucose, with 7 ml of distilled water. This is stored in a dark-coloured glass bottle and can be used for one month. To perform the test, two or three drops of this reagent are added to suspected blood scrapings on a microscope glass slide and preparation covered with a cover slip. After 5 minutes, orange-red/pink feathery crystals characteristic of haemochromogen appear, which are elongated blade-shaped structures of varied sizes joined together at places giving a feathery appearance. Although this test confirms the presence of blood, it does not differentiate between avian and human blood as haemochromogen crystals are seen in both.

Blood Urea Nitrogen : Uric Acid Ratio

Stork[77] reported that BUN/Uric Acid ratio in avian tissue ranges from 1.8:1 to 3.49:1 as compared to a range from 5.52:1 to 27.18:1 in mammalian tissues. In a similar study conducted by Mathur and Adaval,[75] this ratio was found to be 1.8:1 to 2.6:1 in fresh avian blood and 4.5:1 to 5.6:1 in human blood. They also reported that if the samples of blood were exposed to weather conditions like heat, sunlight and dryness, the precipitation of proteins can spuriously lower the values of BUN and Uric Acid. Moreover, to estimate these values on auto-analyzers, a minimum quantity of 125 mg is required, which may be difficult to obtain.

Amino Acid Studies

Emanuel Margoliash of the North Western University and Emil Smith of the University of California at Los Angeles were among the first to notice that the amino acid sequence of various species is different and that the magnitude of the difference corresponds quite well with the distance between the two species on the evolutionary tree. Thus, recent advances in the taxonomy (classification) of animals have resulted from the study of blood proteins and amino acids to determine both interspecies and intraspecies relationships. Amino acid sequence of proteins, particularly nuclear material (DNA), has resulted in reconstructing bird phylogeny (Bird[78] and Sibley[79]).

Species identification is usually carried out by immunological (antigen-antibody) procedures, of which the precipitin test is the most satisfactory. Another technique frequently used for identification of the species of origin employs disc electrophoresis. In this method, the serum or tissue proteins are electrophoretically separated into distinct bands, forming a pattern characteristic of each species (Osler[80], Modi[81]). Serum proteins of turkeys and other domestic fowls were analyzed electrophoreticlly by Flynn and Mayo[82] and results were compared with human serum proteins. They found five fractions with a distribution and relative intensity similar to that found in human serum. Observations of the mobility of protein fractions in fowls suggested that the sera of males in sexually immature birds also separated into five fractions analogous to those of human serum. The albumin fraction in the sera of turkeys and other fowls had a mobility similar to that of man. However, the difference in mobility between beta and gamma globulin was greater in human serum than that of a male in sexually immature fowls and the alpha-2 globulin in fowl serum was slower in comparison with albumin than was the case in human serum.

Schultz et al.[83] used electrophoresis on starch to study amino acids in hydrolyzates of serum proteins. They concluded that proteins of each species could be defined by the distribution of certain amino acids among the electrophoretic components, there being a similarity in distribution among various species in the animal kingdom. La Ham[84] carried out a microscopic examination and amino acid analysis of protein residue obtained from the engine of aircraft known/suspected to have ceased following birdstrikes, for 7 cases. Scrapings from various parts of the aircraft were examined by phase-contrast microscopy. In many cases, fragments of bones and feathers were identifiable. Amino acid analysis was carried out by separation on "chromobeads resins" (Technicon) and the resulting amino acids were automatically plotted on a three-point recorder. La Ham could not obtain an unequivocal amino acid pattern and emphasised the need for a quantitative estimation of amino acids in a greater number of cases.

Since then, amino acid patterns of human and avian blood have been studied by many researchers to explore the possibility of using them as a distinguishing feature in investigations of birdstrike. Amino acid separation has been attempted by thin-layer chromatography. Some researchers have used single and double dimension chromatography and chromatography combined with electrophoresis. Mathur and Adaval[75] used a simple procedure for preparation of specimens, namely, single and double dimension chromatography and the detection of amino acid by staining. They were able to demonstrate six bands of amino acids in avian and human blood samples corresponding to histidine and arginine together, followed by glycine, tyrosine, methionine, phenyl alanine and leucine. Histidine was found to be closest to the point of application. There were no distinct differentiating features except that leucine movement appeared to be marginally greater in avian blood than in human blood. A quantitative study might throw more light on the subject and clarify if these patterns are specific to avian blood. Such estimations can be carried out by an amino-acid-auto-analyzer dedicated for the purpose and a team of trained technical personnel. Samples required for this purpose should be collected under ideal conditions as contamination with any organic or inorganic material may vitiate the results. Thus, the reliability of such estimates in samples collected after air crashes will necessarily be limited.

These procedures may not be useful in aircraft accident investigations, due to the unavailability of blood samples, delay in specimen collection and performance of tests, exposure of samples to air, sunlight, humidity, high temperature and possible contamination by chemical substances. These factors can alter the protein reaction and destroy the capability to combine with specific antibodies. Besides, post-mortem changes introduce numerous artifacts. It has been well established that certain bacteria, like Esch. Coli 096 produce substances identical or very similar to blood group substances and may interfere in immunological procedures of identification. However, DNA typing techniques have since been improved and sophisticated. These may be resorted to in selected cases at assigned laboratories and are not used routinely. In peripheral laboratories, tests like Coomb's Test and ABO blood groups can be performed to detect human blood. In bigger laboratories, absorption-inhibition, absorption-elution, Latte's Crust Test, antiglobulin-inhibition test, interfacial ring-precipitation test, ouchterlony gel double diffusion test etc. may be performed, as advised by Petty and McMeekin.[85]

CHAPTER 7

THE ROLE OF HISTOPATHOLOGY IN FATAL AIR-CRASH INVESTIGATION

Whenever air-crash fatalities are autopsied, the histopathological aspect tends to take a backseat. Injuries are usually so extensive and mutilating that the cause of death appears to be due to "multiple un-survivable injuries". In such circumstances, there is always a tendency to ignore the importance of histopathological investigation. As there is an established procedure for subjecting the tissue to histological examination, routine sampling is sometimes done more to complete the formality than to search for some relevant vital information. This attitude is compounded by the fact that the samples of tissue recovered are in various stages of decomposition either due to delayed retrieval or poor preservation. Thus, a note is often made that "tissue is unsuitable for histological examination".

Some workers have routinely conducted detailed histopathological examinations on air-crash fatalities undaunted by the fact that the cause of accident was obvious. It has gradually become universally accepted that despite the aforementioned discouraging factors, histopathological examination can provide important and valuable information in some (if not all) cases and therefore, must be undertaken with care and precision.[1] When investigating aviation accidents, effects of trauma are to be differentiated from the effects of pre-existing disease. Ante-mortem insult should be segregated from post-crash trauma and injuries should be sequenced to study the chain of events. This is possible only when the pathologist is educated on traumatic histopathology with special reference to air-crash injuries. The importance of some such findings is highlighted below.

Narrowed Coronary Arteries

While conducting histological examination on tissue samples recovered during autopsies, the author has sometimes found a reasonable suspicion of sudden incapacitation of the pilot in charge.[86] A pilot who had collapsed at the controls and died was found to have a haemorrhage in a severely atheromatous coronary artery (Figure 7.1). As the co-pilot managed to land the aircraft safely, the deceased pilot's body was intact and histological findings corroborated the pilot's incapacitation and death at the controls. Had the aircraft crashed, could these findings be incriminated as the cause of the accident? Such clear-cut histopathological findings, which more or less establish the cause of death and even the accident, are few and far between. However, it is worthwhile keeping them in mind while conducting a histological examination.

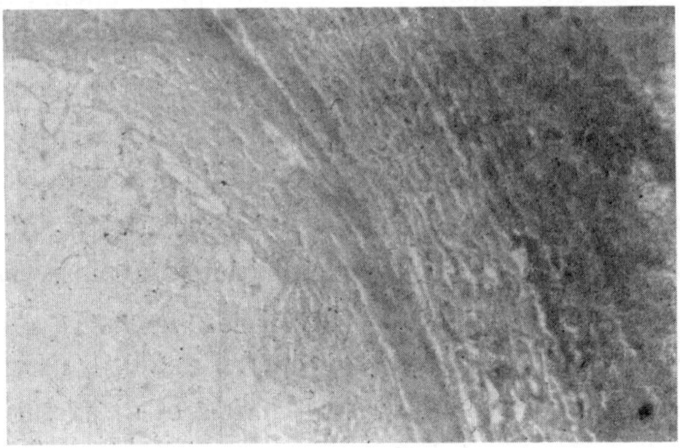

Figure 7.1: Haemorrhage in an atheromatous main coronary artery

Some findings encountered during histopathological examination reveal conditions which could cause sudden incapacitation of the pilot. An autopsy conducted on a pilot showed more than 90 per cent narrowing of the left anterior descending coronary artery (Figure 7.2) and 70–75 per cent narrowing of the other two main vessels. Associated fatty changes of a severe degree were also found in the liver. With such compromised coronary circulation, there is always a possibility of sudden spasm of one of these blood vessels, leading to arrhythmia and even sudden cardiac standstill. Thus, due consideration must be given to such findings. The accident may or may not have occurred due to the pilot's incapacitation, but it is the duty of the pathologist to point out these findings to other investigating authorities who can evaluate them in the light of circumstantial evidence.

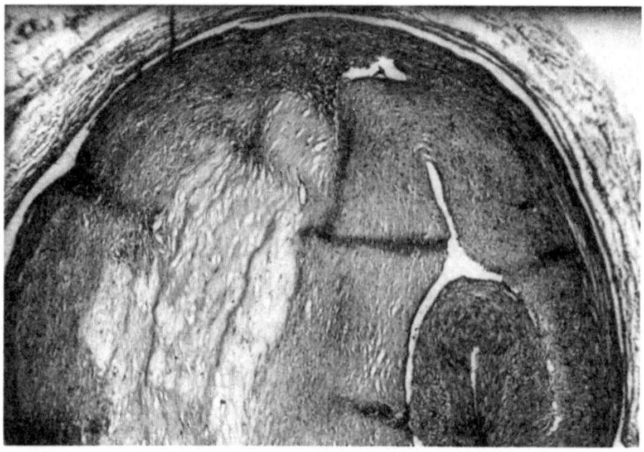

Figure 7.2: Section of left anterior descending coronary artery with extreme narrowing of lumen

As the incidence of coronary artery disease is increasing in younger age groups, such findings in a pilot assume significance. This is particularly true when no other cause of accident is found. Some pilots, who are known to have suffered from anginal pain in-flight, have nevertheless managed to land safely. Upon investigation, these pilots were found to have suffered from acute episodes of Ischemic Heart Disease (IHD).[87] On the other hand, many fatal accidents have been attributed to this condition. Stevens[2] described an accident in which 83 persons were killed due to the pilot's incapacitation from IHD. Buley[88] recorded four such cases. Townsend[27] reported on a case of sudden death of a co-pilot while flying. In 9 fatal accidents, Glantz and Stembridge[89] found extensive atherosclerotic process in coronary arteries, severely narrowing their lumen. In these cases, the investigating authorities could not find the exact cause of the accident and the pilot's incapacitation continued to be considered a possible causal factor. At US AFIP, Townsend and Glantz[90] found at least 6 cases in which there was a definite possibility of the accident having been caused due to coronary episodes. Rayman[91] analyzed such cases of myocardial infarction in pilots during a 10-year period and found at least 2 confirmed and 5 doubtful cases of in-flight episodes. Adaval et al.[92] and Tunstall-Pedoe H[93] have mentioned that fatal accident rates in passenger aircraft can be compared directly with coronary heart attack rates in pilots. These authors concluded that, although "heart attacks" can occur suddenly and can cause incapacitation of a pilot, a very small percentage of accidents is actually attributable to them. They also point out that pilots should be at lower risk than the general population of the same age group due to frequent medical checks and the fact that persons with very early evidence of coronary artery disease may not be allowed to fly. In this context, it is relevant to note that Fechner and Sivaloganathan[94] have highlighted studies under fluorescence microscope to detect the presence of myocardial infarction in putrefying bodies, which can be useful for an aviation pathologist under certain circumstances.

The pathologist should not be carried away by these findings and jump to the conclusion that accidents are attributable to in-flight coronary episodes. It is well documented that severely narrowed coronary arteries may just be coincidental findings. At the same time, sudden death or incapacitation may occur even when there is no histological evidence of thrombosis or haemorrhage.[2] Thus, Scheiman[95] has advised caution in implicating narrowed coronary arteries in the pilot-in-charge as the cause of accident.

Focal Myocarditis

Another condition that can be responsible for a pilot's sudden incapacitation is "focal myocarditis". The author investigated a case in which an experienced pilot was practising a close air-support manoeuvre. The aircraft pulled up, went into a steep dive and crashed, killing the pilot. No technical snag was found in the aircraft and the cause of accident was attributed to "pilot error" or human failure. An autopsy was performed, despite fragmentation of the body. Only a small piece of heart muscle was recovered, which was totally embedded in 16 paraffin blocks. A thorough histological study of slides prepared from all these blocks showed unmistakable lesions of focal myocarditis (Figure 7.3) in two such blocks (Adaval et al.[96]).

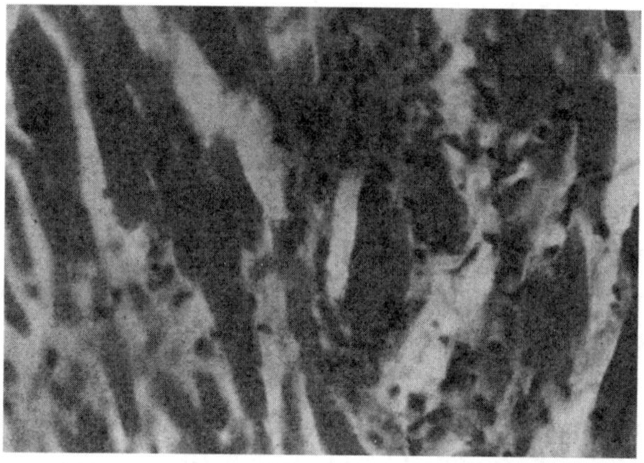

Figure 7.3: Lesion of focal myocarditis in one of the histological sections

This finding stimulated discussion on focal myocarditis vis-à-vis sudden death in an apparently healthy individual — a fact well recognised by forensic pathologists. It is also known that focal myocarditis may be encountered incidentally in about 5 per cent of cases in which the cause of death is totally unrelated to the cardiovascular system (e.g. mechanical trauma). As histological evidence of focal myocarditis may be encountered frequently by an aviation pathologist, it will always be a source of confusion as to whether it caused sudden incapacitation of the pilot or was a mere incidental finding. Consequently, a few paragraphs need to be devoted to this subject.

In 1837, Sobernhein introduced this condition into medical literature. Later, in 1890, Fiedler described it in relation to myocardial involvement. Since then, myocarditis has been given several names like Isolated, Fiedler's idiopathic, Primary Acute Interstitial and Focal/Diffuse Myocarditis. According to Saphir,[97] myocarditis can be categorized as: (a) post-infection (with or without involvement of the endocardium), (b) disease-specific (tubercular or rheumatic etc.), (c) post-traumatic (physical or chemical) and (d) isolated (where there is no associated disease anywhere in the body).

Focal (isolated) myocarditis is of greatest interest to the aviation pathologist. As there are no associated systemic lesions, this condition may be encountered during an autopsy of a pilot who was apparently healthy and fit to fly. Therefore, the definition of this lesion and its histological criteria has been discussed in detail by Stevens and Underwood Ground.[98] They recommended that focal inflammatory infiltrate (with/without muscle necrosis) that is not associated with any systemic disease or pathology elsewhere should be the criterion. The quantum of inflammatory cells was fixed at approximately 100 or more if only a single lesion was encountered. If there was more than one focus, any lesion of about half this size was taken as significant. During the 7th Scientific Session of the Joint Committee of Aviation Pathology (JCAP) in 1969, the same criteria were discussed and endorsed. Because this yardstick has been established, it has become necessary for a pathologist to look for these lesions in histological sections of myocardial tissue. The greater the amount of tissue studied, the greater is the chance of finding these lesions. It is recommended by Adaval et al.[96] that while taking samples from the deceased pilot's heart when investigating a fatal air crash, care must be exercised to examine a large number of sections representing a substantial portion of the myocardium and not restrict the study to just one or two sections, especially when pilot incapacitation is suspected.

Focal (isolated) myocarditis has been considered by many workers to cause sudden death in an apparently healthy individual. The mechanism described is sudden arrhythmia generated by an inflammatory focus near the conduction system (self-electrocution!). It is suspected that ventricular arrhythmia initiated from a focus of myocarditis may produce ventricular fibrillation and even failure. Although myocarditis is frequently secondary to many pathological conditions, its presence in an apparently healthy person, who is suspected to having become suddenly incapacitated, should be taken seriously. Though the general incidence of focal myocarditis in forensic autopsies is quite low, it is as high as 14 per cent when no other acceptable cause of death is found.[98–101]

A pathologist should keep this condition in mind while helping other investigating authorities. A pilot's medical history may be clean, as the presence of focal myocarditis can go undetected during a routine ECG examination. When no obvious cause of accident is discovered on the basis of findings of other investigating channels, the total circumstances of the accident are reviewed, and pilot error or human failure is often incriminated. A finding of focal myocarditis at this stage should be highlighted by the pathologist and its implications explained, especially to non-medical authorities. It is important to point out that although this condition can be just a coincidental finding, it can also produce sudden incapacitation, even death.

Fatty Liver

An autopsy of an air-signaller, who died in an aircraft accident (totally unrelated to the cause of accident) revealed moderate atheromatous coronary arteries but extensive fatty changes in the liver (Figure 7.4). Besides this, early cirrhotic changes were also found to have set in. Although severe fatty changes in the liver may not have any relation to accident causation, it is interesting to note that some workers have attributed sudden death to a fatty liver. Persons with fatty livers are known to react adversely to decompression and to have a high incidence of fat embolism and increased vulnerability to toxic hazards. They are also more prone to hypoglycaemia.

When a fatty liver is encountered, the pathologist should classify it as mild, moderate or severe, as done by Townsend and Glantz[90] and Mason.[1] Although there may be rare cases of pilot incapacitation due to fatty liver, this condition is important as it throws light on poor general health. Adaval and Kunzru[86] have found severe fatty changes in 10 per cent of cases and in

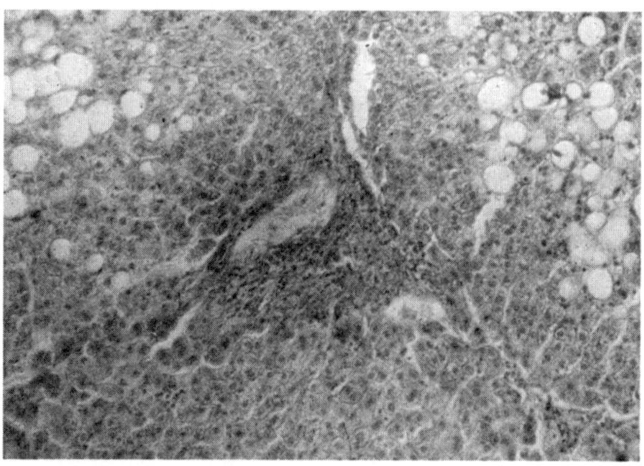

Figure 7.4: Marked fatty changes in liver with evidence of early fibrosis

all of them there were associated moderate to severe atheromatous changes in the coronary arteries. Though not directly responsible for accident, these findings show poor health of a pilot and a possible habit of heavy drinking, particularly when encountered in a younger age group.

Fat and Bone Marrow Embolism

Some findings are extremely valuable in reconstructing the chain of events during and after an aircraft accident. While trying to do this, it becomes necessary to time the injuries and put them in chronological order as far as possible. This task is very difficult, and at times impossible, because of the very short time interval involved. To quote a simple example, if there is an injury to the occupant during flight (e.g. fracture, burns), its evidence will be lost if the aircraft crashed immediately thereafter. The victim's body will show extensive trauma and post-crash burns and it will be impossible to segregate ante-mortem injuries from trauma that is sustained during terminal impact. Thus, during medical reconstruction, it is often difficult to tell which injury occurred earlier. Histological evidence of cellular response around bruises and contusions has been of little help because of the short time interval involved between causation of injury and cessation of circulation. Haemorrhagic and bloodless fractures in the same body have provided some valuable clues, as highlighted earlier. In this context, "the embolic phenomenon" is of great help wherein pulmonary fat and bone marrow embolism are of value in sequencing the injuries. Thus, an aviation pathologist must study this phenomenon in great detail.

Fat Embolism

Warthin[102] long ago emphasised the importance of tissue embolism vis-à-vis ante-mortem trauma. Though Lehman and Moore[103] expressed some reservations about this, it was generally accepted that injury to fat depots of the body produced fat embolism if circulation was intact. After the violence, the fat cell envelope ruptures and if veins are torn along with a localised increase in pressure, fat enters into the blood circulation (Gauss[104]). Of course, circulation of blood should necessarily continue to enable these emboli to travel and be deposited elsewhere.

The embolic phenomenon has been studied by a number of workers.[105–110] After Armstrong et al.[6] published their report on Comet disasters, however, the real value of the embolic phenomenon in reconstructing events and sequencing injuries came to be appreciated. Later, this subject was studied in greater detail by Hickey and Stembridge[111] and Mason.[112,113] Its importance in air-crash investigation was soon realised, due to several comprehensive studies. Mason[1] classified pulmonary fat embolism based upon the ease with which it is found in histological sections of lungs. According to him, incidence of pulmonary fat embolism was much higher in cases of death due to ground accidents than in cases of aircraft accidents. Obviously, this is due to the fact that trauma in air crashes is too sudden and extensive and does not permit time for emboli to develop due to sudden cessation of circulation. Thus, the greater the ferocity and extent of trauma, the less the evidence of embolism.

In the lungs, emboli are distributed uniformly. There is no predilection for any lobe or area. Therefore, when embolism is suspected, a large portion of lung tissue should be processed for histological examination. Similarly, it is not established whether a fracture or trauma to any particular bone is more likely than a fracture to another to produce these emboli. In deaths due to extensive trauma and multiple fractures, pulmonary emboli may not be found, due to sudden death. At the same time, fat embolism develops at great speed and if circulation is intact for even a very short time, emboli find their way into the lungs.[111] Even mild to moderate trauma to subcutaneous fat (as encountered during ejection from an aircraft or in decompression) can cause some amount of pulmonary fat embolism. Buchnan[114] has mentioned that sometimes even a procedure like resuscitation (artificial respiration) to a patient can produce fat and even bone marrow embolism. Busuttil[115] has described an interactive semi-automated procedure of quantitative determination of volume of fat emboli in tissue using image analysis. This procedure was developed to obtain reliable and reproducible data for epidemiological purposes, especially in air-crash fatalities, and to correlate the findings with other injuries, such as bone fractures and severe trauma.

If an individual survives for a longer time after sustaining the trauma, more and more fat embolism builds in. Small chylo-microns are instantly seen in the blood and these coalesce to form bigger particles. The big particles then get deposited in the lungs (Figure 7.5). A high concentration of emboli can therefore be seen in "hours" rather than "minutes". It is not necessary to expect fracture of bones if only fat embolism is found. Adaval et al.[24] have graded the survival of air-crash casualties in "seconds", "minutes" and "hours", based upon the quantum of fat emboli found in the lungs. They recommend that importance be given to moderately and markedly positive cases, where competence of circulation and survival time can be assessed with some degree of certainty and, therefore, early retrieval and processing of large amounts of lung tissue is necessary.

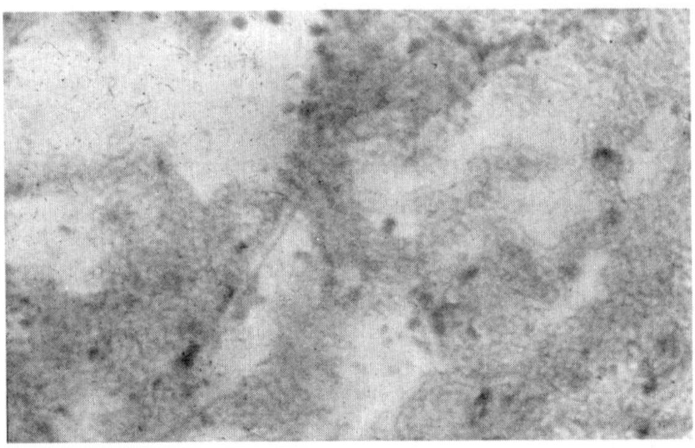

Figure 7.5: Section of lung, markedly positive for fat emboli

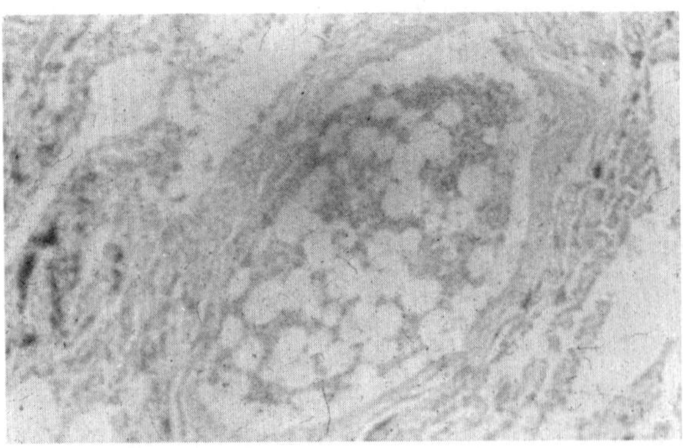

Figure 7.6: Histological section of lung showing a bone marrow embolus

Figure 7.6 shows a bone marrow embolus in a section of lung. The deceased was a pilot who had sustained multiple deceleration trauma, including fractures of several bones and survived only for a few minutes after sustaining this trauma. Fat emboli were also found in the lung tissue.

Bone marrow embolism in the lungs also denotes ante-mortem trauma to bones. It is encountered less often than fat emboli and can sometimes be difficult to detect, especially in poorly preserved tissue. Bierre[116] has reported on the post-mortem examination of 231 victims of an Air New Zealand DC 10 air crash. In this case, pulmonary fat embolism was found in 134 (65 per cent) and pulmonary bone marrow embolism in 60 (29 per cent) cases. A clear relationship was found between the extent of fat and bone marrow embolism, their association with pulmonary oedema and severity of cardiovascular damage. Adaval and Kunzru[24,86] compared bone marrow and fat embolic phenomenon in "immediate death group" and found that half of the cases with fat embolism showed bone marrow embolism as well. When individuals lived for "hours" after trauma, the likelihood of finding bone marrow embolism declined sharply, whereas fat embolism became more severe and frequent. This is due to the resolution of bone marrow embolism, which is rapid and begins in about 6 hours, when venous emboli may start appearing. This aspect throws additional light on survival time vis-à-vis rescue operations and also has a medico-legal bearing on the relative survival of different individuals who are subjected to the same hostile environment.

Thus, both types of emboli appear in seconds — soon after trauma— but fat emboli are faster to arise. With time (if the individual survives), fat embolism increases quantitatively to reach a peak in 4 to 5 days whereas marrow embolism undergoes resolution after about 6 hours and may appear as venous emboli a few hours thereafter. In spite of the differences in the incidence, there is no doubt that both types indicate ante-mortem trauma and provide useful clues for timing and sequencing the injuries.

Although some histological findings may not help to establish the cause of accident or the sequencing of injuries, they nevertheless provide useful knowledge of traumatic pathology. Many such findings may be confused with those encountered in organic lesions and, therefore, a pathologist must familiarise himself with such pictures.

Traumatic Pneumonosis and Emphysema

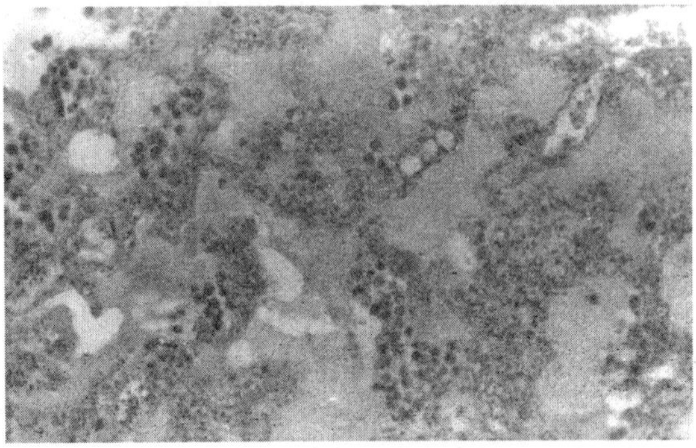

Figure 7.7: Histological section of lung showing extruded alveolar phagocytes in the alveolar spaces

Figure 7.7 shows a section from the lungs of an air-crash victim who died of multiple violent injuries. In such deceleration injuries, it is not uncommon to find a histological picture of "traumatic pneumonosis". Here, there is extrusion of alveolar phagocytes, which now lie in the alveolar spaces. Appearance may range from sparse scattering of phagocytes resembling "heart failure cells" to aggregates of these cells in large numbers, which may fill up the alveolus. These cells are carbon-containing macrophages torn off from alveolar septae or bronchioles due to violent trauma. Figure 7.8 shows such phagocytes lying in the bronchiolar lumen.

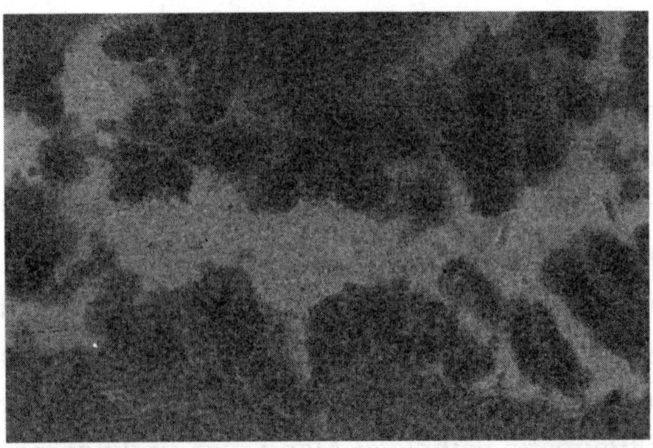

Figure 7.8: Alveolar phagocytes in bronchiolar lumen

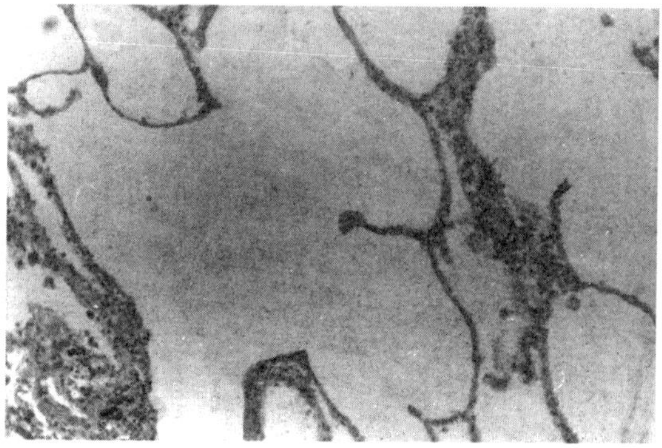

Figure7.9: Histological section of lung showing broken alveolar walls

Figure 7.9 highlights a typical picture of "traumatic emphysema". When traumatic emphysema is present without collapse, it is usually manifest to the greatest extent in the sub-pleural region. In most cases, the appearance of a traumatically broken alveolar wall is histologically different from the picture of clinical emphysema. As seen in Figure 7.9, the broken wall has a blunted end, which is absent in organic emphysema. Moreover, associated findings such as traumatic pneumonosis, a predilection to sub-pleural areas, and alternating areas of collapse and emphysema will easily differentiate it from that of clinical emphysema.

From the examples provided in this chapter, it is evident that histological findings in relation to fatal aircraft accidents fall into four groups. According to Adaval and Kunzru[86] the first group includes findings that more or less establish the cause of the accident. The second includes features that are of doubtful value as far as cause of accident is concerned but point out a certain possibility (like the pilot's sudden incapacitation). The third group contains findings that are helpful in timing and sequencing of injuries and help in working out the chain of events during and after the accident. The fourth group includes histological features that provide insight into traumatic pathology especially in relation to aviation accidents. Aviation pathologists are advised to carry out meticulous and painstaking histological examinations and build a databank. Areas of future research include those which provide evidence of earliest cellular response to injury and changes in adrenals associated with sudden stress.

CHAPTER 8

COLLECTION AND STORAGE OF SPECIMENS

In all aircraft accidents, it is necessary to determine whether the aircrew became incapacitated before or during the accident. This incapacitation could be due to a pre-existing disease or to a toxic environment either inside the body (e.g. the action of certain drugs/alcohol) or outside (fire, fumes, smoke, carbon monoxide, hypoxia, etc.). Therefore, the collection of biological samples during autopsies is necessary, even if the cause of death and accident is very obvious on the basis of other evidence. It is the duty of the pathologist performing the autopsy to ensure proper collection, preservation, storage and dispatch of such samples. Some useful tips for this procedure are detailed below.

Specimens for Histological Studies

Pieces from all available organs should be preserved for histological examination as soon after the death as possible. Tissues from suspected sites of disease and burns, skin, brain, liver, kidneys, spleen, oesophagus, stomach, trachea, adrenal glands, pancreas, bronchi and all lobes of both lungs should always be preserved. Substantial lung tissue should be sampled, if possible, as the processing required for detecting fat and bone marrow embolism must be undertaken using these samples. Stomach contents may be preserved as they are useful in timing the death (state of digestion of food) and also for detection of drugs/alcohol. The heart should be preserved as a whole. For better preservation, it is necessary to open the chambers. Cutting open the heart along its whole right and left borders is sufficient. Unless the autopsy is performed by an aviation pathology expert, the coronary arteries should not be cut or probed.

Generally, 1cm thick pieces of tissue, each weighing approximately 150 to 200 gm are adequate. Smaller organs should be taken in full and later sliced as required. When dismembered and mutilated bodies are encountered, tissues from whatever organs/sites are available, should be preserved for histological study. A state of decomposition and mutilation should not deter a pathologist from collection of these samples. Very useful information can often be obtained from even putrefied samples. A checklist of the sites from where tissue is to be collected is provided below:

Brain

Cerebrum: Coronal section

Cerebellum: Coronal section

Midbrain, pons, medulla oblongata

Look for contusion of the medulla, which may be encountered when there is a whiplash movement of the head on the cervical spine.

In addition to the routine collection of tissue, remove any part of the brain that looks suspicious of any pathology. Take portions of the brain if they show any contusion or haemorrhage and note the correlation of this injury with external trauma if any, e.g. fractures of the skull bones.

Pituitary Gland

Preserve as a whole.

Thyroid Gland

Take a 2cm x 1cm section from each lobe and isthmus. This is to rule out any pathology like goitre or hyperthyroidism.

Respiratory Tract

Pieces of trachea and bronchi

In the case of fire, the entire trachea and bronchial tree should be preserved for a detailed examination. If soot particles are encountered, their exact position should be noted and the soot particles should be preserved in a separate container, without any added preservative. The study of soot particles is very useful in detecting the origin and nature of the fire.

Lungs

Pieces from each lobe of the lungs are ideal. However, if only a part of the lung tissue is available, a substantial amount may be preserved. This tissue, besides being used for routine histopathological examination, will also be needed to study fat and bone-marrow embolism.

Heart and Great Blood Vessels

Pieces from great blood vessels may be taken, keeping in mind the vulnerability of certain areas to deceleration trauma. Routine samples are also required in order to study atheromatous changes.

Preserve the heart as a whole for detailed study later. For fixation, cut open along its right and left borders. Coronary arteries can be studied in detail after fixation.

Abdomen

Pieces from the stomach, and small and large intestines are important. The liver should be examined for areas of rupture and haemorrhage and sampled accordingly. Even if no macroscopic pathology is noted, it is prudent to collect tissue from the liver for "routine" histopathology. Gross fatty changes are frequently encountered in the liver and generally indicate the health of the pilot. They also provide evidence of chronic alcoholism and vulnerability to explosive decompression illness. Routine histopathology of the pancreas may show changes suggestive of diabetes mellitus. Kidneys may be preserved in the form of slices from both sides. A study is currently in progress to determine histological changes in the adrenal glands during acute stress and so it is worthwhile to collect them in total. The spleen may be examined to detect areas of rupture and haemorrhage and sampled accordingly.

Lymph Nodes

Abnormally enlarged lymph nodes may be collected and sliced

immediately. This is to rule out the possibility of pre-existing disease.

Skin

In cases of burns, burnt skin as well as adjoining normal skin should be preserved in its whole thickness. The entire skin should be carefully examined and if any powdering/peppering is found, the same should be preserved for histological as well as toxicological purposes. Careful noting of the site from where the skin piece is removed should be documented, preferably with the help of a sketch diagram.

Containers

Self-sealing .005 gauge polythene bags, 22x37 cm in size, are satisfactory for routine use. They are easy to handle, reasonably priced, occupy relatively less space and are convenient to transport. Alternatively, wide mouth plastic screw-capped bottles with a 0.5–2.0 litre capacity may be adequate.

Preservatives

The preservative for histopathological study is 10 per cent formal-saline. This can be kept ready or may be prepared fresh at the time of autopsy. For an "on-the-spot autopsy", it is convenient to carry polythene bags (22x37cm size) which can contain about 400 ml of formal-saline. Accurately measured quantities of formalin and sodium chloride can be kept in small containers and, when required, can be mixed with tap-water in a polythene container to get the required strength of preservative solution. A mixture of 40 ml of formalin, 3.6 gm of sodium chloride and 360 ml (3/4-full polythene bag) of tap-water will produce the required 400 ml of formal-saline. To ensure proper fixation, the tissue should be suitably sliced to allow the preservative to penetrate. The volume of the preservative should be approximately 8 to 10 times the volume of the tissue to be preserved.

Storage

Once the preservative has been added to the tissues, the specimens can be kept at room temperature. No refrigeration is required.

Samples for Biochemical and Toxicological Studies

It is current practice in the case of fatal aircraft accidents to conduct biochemical/toxicological tests on the deceased aircrew. These tests provide estimates of blood ethanol (alcohol), carboxyhaemoglobin and brain lactic acid (only when hypoxia is suspected). The presence of drugs and other toxic agents is determined when circumstantial evidence warrants. Routine studies and body fluid/tissues required are indicated below:-

STUDY	TISSUE/BODY FLUID
Lactic acid estimation (only in cases where hypoxia is suspected)	Brain/Kidney/Blood
Ethanol (ethyl alcohol)	Blood/Urine/Liver tissue extract/vitreous humour

Collection of Samples

Lactic Acid

For brain lactic acid estimation, about 150 gm of sliced brain is collected as soon after the death as possible. Polythene bags of the sort suggested for collecting histological specimens can be used here as well. After closing (knotting) a bag, it must be immediately frozen under ice in a thermos flask or in the freezing compartment of a refrigerator. Dry ice (carbon dioxide snow) is the ideal freezing agent if it is available. No preservative should be used and the tissue should be kept in a frozen state continuously during storage and transit until estimation is complete.

For blood lactic acid estimation, 5 ml of blood should be collected in sodium fluoride (10 mg of sodium fluoride per ml of blood) and preserved in either a small well-stoppered sterile bottle or in unmedicated condoms, which can be closed by knotting. (Rubber condoms can be sterilised and stored in the same way as surgical gloves.) Sodium fluoride should be properly mixed with the sample. The specimen should be stored and transited in frozen state.

Ethanol

Five ml each of blood or urine is preserved with sodium fluoride (10 mg per ml of fluid) and can be collected in sterile screw-capped bottles or condoms. Storage and transit should be in the same way as in the case of samples for lactic acid.

Carbon Monoxide

Blood and muscle tissue are collected and preserved in frozen state, without any chemical or preservative. Muscle tissue can be collected in the same manner as brain tissue for lactic acid determination. Approximately 100 gm of muscle tissue in polythene bags and 20 ml of blood in sterile screw-capped bottles or condoms would be adequate. Storage and transmission should be done in frozen state, as for lactic acid determination.

Drugs

Specimens like blood, urine, stomach contents and tissue extracts are collected and kept frozen without adding any preservatives unless specified otherwise. If a preservative is added at all, a sample of the same preservative should invariably be saved and kept along with the specimen collected for use as a control. If possible, the urine sample should be collected by puncturing the urinary bladder with a needle attached to a syringe under sterile conditions. The sample of blood from the heart should be taken in the same way.

Recommendations from a USAF Flight Surgeon's Guide

The USAF Flight Surgeon's Guide[34] specifies that when samples are required from survivors of the accident, 15–20 ml of serum (without preservative), 15–20 ml of blood with sodium fluoride, the same amount of blood with EDTA, and 70 ml of urine without preservative is sufficient. In cases of fatalities, 100 ml of blood, 100 ml of urine without preservatives, bile and vitreous humour (if available), 100–200 gm brain, 50 gm kidney and 50 gm lung tissue is recommended along with 50 gm gastric contents. Regarding the requirement of dry ice, nearly double the weight of dry ice is required vis-à-vis the weight of tissue when transportation is likely to take up to 72 hours and ambient temperature is up to 100°F. When this temperature is over 100 degrees, the time of transit should not exceed 48 hours and tissue:dry ice ratio should be increased to 1:6.

Labelling of Samples

The following information should be legibly written with waterproof ink and attached to the specimen. (Sometimes, it is also useful to slip this label between two polyethylene bags):

Name of deceased
Autopsy/Body Number
Date & Time of death/accident
Date & Time of collection of specimen
Nature of specimen
Name of preservative — if used

CHAPTER 9

AUTOPSY EQUIPMENT

Speed and mobility is of utmost importance in conducting a good autopsy in air-crash situations. Consequently, the pathologist who is likely to be entrusted with this task should remain in a state of instant readiness. The equipment required for an autopsy, suitable containers and all other necessary materials must be kept ready at all times. It is, therefore, advisable to have a portable autopsy kit which can be taken to the site of accident for "on-the-spot" autopsies. The necessary equipment, including the components of this kit, is listed below:

1. Autopsy Equipment
   Post-mortem saw
   Belfast rib-shearer 31 cm
   Knife ligament 37 cm
   Blowpipe
   Chisel
   Knife handles sizes 3 & 4 with suitable blades
   Organ knife 18 cm
   Brain knife
   Cartilage knife
   Viscera knife 25 cm
   Scissors, bowel
   Scissors, dressing, straight with both points sharp, 12.5 cm
   Chisel with detachable cross handle
   Electric saw

Tissue micro-magnifier
Hammer & chisel, combined 22 cm
Coronet
Hooks, sharp with chain sets
Spirit lamp
Rubber gloves
Disposable aprons, masks
Plastic aprons
Rubber boots
Measuring tape
Disposable sterile syringes of various sizes, 2 ml to 20 ml
Plastic collection bags
Packets of pre-weighed sodium chloride
Sodium fluoride bottle
Wide-mouthed thermos flask, 5-litre capacity
Weighing balance, 5-kg capacity
Writing material, papers, glass marking pencil, clips, stamp pad
Suture material including curved needles
Absorbent cotton rolls
Fibre-glass container, autopsy equipment carriage bag
Charts for polar and wreckage scatter diagrams

2. Toxicology specimen containers

3. Formalin specimen containers

Recommended contents of portable autopsy kit:

A. Folding autopsy table with attachments for instrument tray, water flushing device, portable battery-operated flashlights and camera
B. Autopsy instrument box containing:
    (a) Scalpels
    (b) Knives — organ, brain, ligaments, dissecting, visceral/brain, cartilage
    (c) Scissors

(d) Saws
(e) Chisel and hammer
(f) Rib-shearers
(g) Blowpipe
(h) Forceps
(i) Hooks, needles, suture material
(j) Absorbent cotton
(k) Battery-operated electrical saw
(l) Tissue micro magnifier
(m) Spirit lamp
(n) Gloves
(o) Disposable aprons
(p) Disposable masks
(q) Measuring tape
(r) Disposable syringes
(s) Suture material
(t) Formalin pure in plastic bottles
(u) Packets of pre-weighed sodium chloride
(v) Wide-mouthed thermos flasks
(w) Sodium fluoride, pre-weighed
(x) Polythene collection bags of various sizes, self-sealing type
(y) Miscellaneous items, such as:
Writing paper
Dot pens
Glass-marking pencils
Charts
Clip/Flags
Charts for polar diagrams
Charts for wreckage-distribution diagrams
Fibreglass containers of various sizes
Portable weighing scale to weigh up to 5 kg
Autopsy equipment carriage bag
Toxicology specimen container
Histopathology specimen container

Camera with flashlight
Checklist for observations to be made during autopsy
Soap and disposable hand towels
Rubber-shoes (gum boots)

CHAPTER 10

SOME INSTANCES

During my stint of more than 20 years in the field of Aviation Accident Pathology, having been inducted from the discipline of Clinical Pathology to this specialised field, I had to gradually learn about this discipline from senior specialists and also through my own experience. This experience included many instances of not only success, but also "missed opportunities" and "shortfalls". Facts and figures in the following examples may not be very accurate, as the details of these investigations are being recalled from memory. However, these examples highlight the general principles of Aviation Accident Pathology, as defined by Mason[1].

Investigation 1

As a young pathologist, almost totally ignorant of the intricacies of this specialised field, sometime in 1968, I was called upon to perform an autopsy on the body of an experienced pilot who ejected from a Canberra aircraft and was found dead in a field. Forensic authorities had readily authorized a pathologist from the Armed Forces to do the necessary work as the aircraft and pilot belonged to the Air Force and no civilian casualties or property was involved.

Armed with knowledge of General Pathology, I set about my task meticulously. I was surprised to note that the pilot's body was more or less intact, except for a few minor abrasions and contusions here and there. X-rays of all bones revealed no fractures. The internal organs were intact and thus the cause of death was not obvious. Unable to solve this riddle, I requested the higher authorities to call a senior aviation pathologist who could help me out. Fortunately, the senior pathologist arrived the same day. "Do not work in isolation," he advised. "Let us go and talk with other teams who are investigating this accident simultaneously."

We learned from further discussions that this was a "through canopy ejection" where the canopy of the aircraft is broken when the pilot bales out through it. This information led us to look for injury especially in the head/neck region. Meticulous dissection revealed an anterior fracture of first cervical vertebra with corresponding haemorrhages in the brain stem and spinal cord. The pattern looked as if the head was forced into hyper-extension at atlanto-occipital junction. Inspection of the helmet did not reveal any damage or scratches.

The injury to bony structures was not discernible in X-rays because the head had returned to its original position, and because of interposition of soft tissues. (This is the reason why we now recommend that a lateral view of occipital-first cervical junction should be taken with the head under 25 pounds of traction).

In the light of this new finding, we attempted to reconstruct the sequence of events in this accident in consultation with specialists of other groups. In the beginning, things appeared to be quite simple. The cause of this cervical injury was attributed to through-canopy-ejection when the pilot's neck was not held in an ideal position. However, something was amiss. We relentlessly continued to look into other factors, examining the ejection seat, life-support system and parachute. We soon struck pay dirt. That is, the pilot had pulled the 'D' ring. This ring is pulled manually when the parachute does not deploy automatically. This, indirectly, meant that after the ejection sequence, the parachute did not open automatically and the pilot tried to open it manually by pulling the 'D' ring. At the same time, it is also almost certain that a person with injury of such severity at the brain stem and cervical spine would have quadruplegia (paralysis of all limbs) and would be unable to move his arms at all, let alone pulling the 'D' ring! This meant that the spinal injury must have occurred after the 'D' ring was pulled, during the descent phase of parachute landing.

An examination of the parachute showed that there was faulty deployment that could throw a pilot into a spin in mid-air. A re-examination of the body showed a significant deep linear abrasion over the area between chin and throat which conformed to the pattern of rig lines of parachute.

We, therefore, concluded that the pilot had successfully ejected through the canopy without sustaining any injury during this phase. During descent, as the parachute did not deploy automatically, he pulled the 'D' ring. Due to faulty deployment, a rig line of the parachute got under the neck and forced his head in hyperextension, resulting in the injuries to the spine and sudden death.

Five lessons were learned from this investigation:

(a) A pathologist should not work in isolation and must interact with other teams that are simultaneously investigating the accident.

(b) He should thoroughly familiarise himself with circumstances of accident, aircraft involved and its life-support system.

(c) Ordinary X-rays may not show minor damage to bones such as cracks or green-stick fractures because of the interposition of soft tissue. When suspected, the bone has to be examined and X-rays repeated after the soft tissue is removed.

(d) An X-ray of occipital-first cervical junction of neck should be taken with head under 25 pounds of traction.

(e) Experience, logical deductive reasoning and an open mind have their own value. One should not hesitate to seek help from an experienced aviation pathologist as it may be just a matter of "what one knows — one sees!"

Investigation 2

In the early 1970s, at an airbase in the Eastern Sector of India, on a clear starry night, two young flyers prepared for a leisurely practice of night flying in a Dakota aircraft — an old war-horse transport aircraft (Figure 10.1). After an "all clear", the engine was started and an instrument check was performed. Suddenly, the pilot in-charge told his co-pilot that he suspected an engine leak. He let the engine run, took a hand torchlight and came out of the aircraft. The co-pilot kept sitting in the cockpit and watched his friend facing the aircraft and flashing the torchlight towards engines.

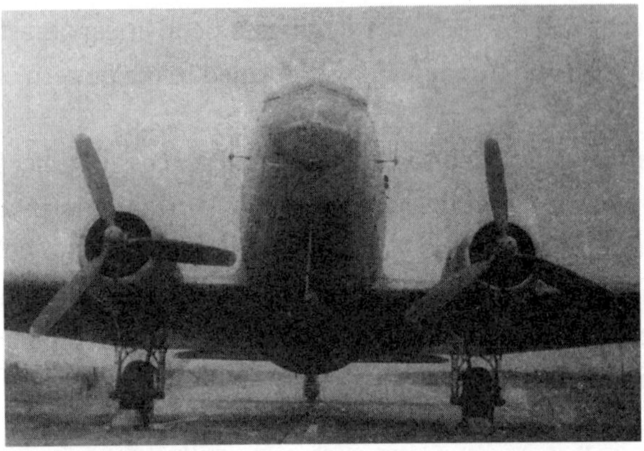

Figure 10.1: A Dakota transport aircraft on the runway

Suddenly, a loud thud was heard and the co-pilot could see the body of his leader hurled into the air. He switched off the engines and yelled for help. Within minutes, the entire area was cordoned off. Ambulance, paramedics, a medical doctor and others arrived. The pilot's body was lying a few yards from the engines but his head and left arm were missing. Further search recovered these parts. It appeared as if the head was severed from the torso at the level of the upper neck and left arm at the level of the axilla. These parts, along with the main trunk, were removed and preserved at the mortuary.

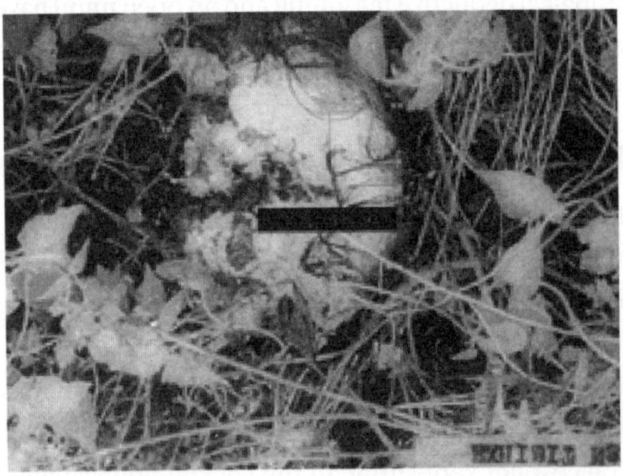

Figure 10.2: Severed head lying a few yards from the aircraft

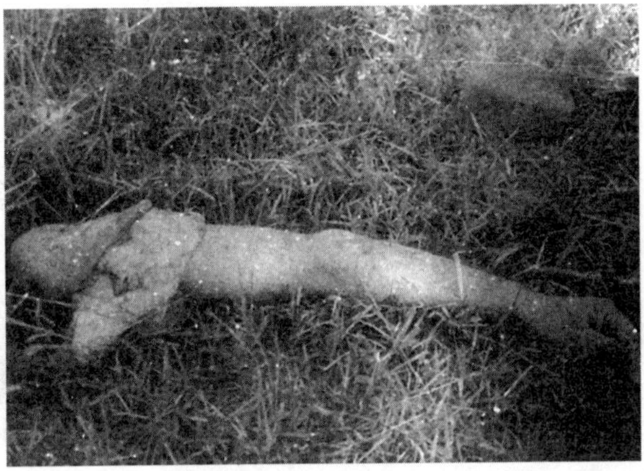

Figure 10.3: Left arm lying a few yards away from the aircraft

The next day, I was called to perform the autopsy. The body had been preserved on ice, with all clothing removed and kept aside. Before beginning the autopsy, the circumstances of accident were explained to me. I was told that this was a clear-cut case of the pilot walking into propeller blades, as he misjudged the distance between himself and the blades in the dark. The autopsy confirmed two significant features. The left upper extremity (arm, forearm and hand) was severed from the main trunk at the level of the axilla. The head was separated from the trunk at the upper part of neck. However, there was also a slash at the top part of the head, removing a part of vault of skull and overlying scalp. (The pilot had removed his helmet before getting down from the aircraft.)

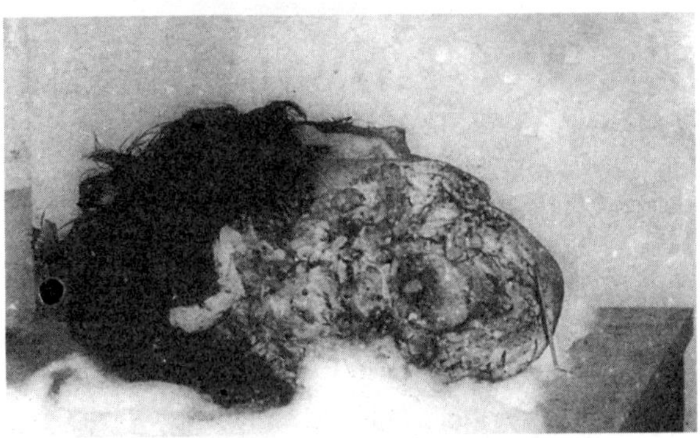

Figure 10.4: Head separated from upper part of neck

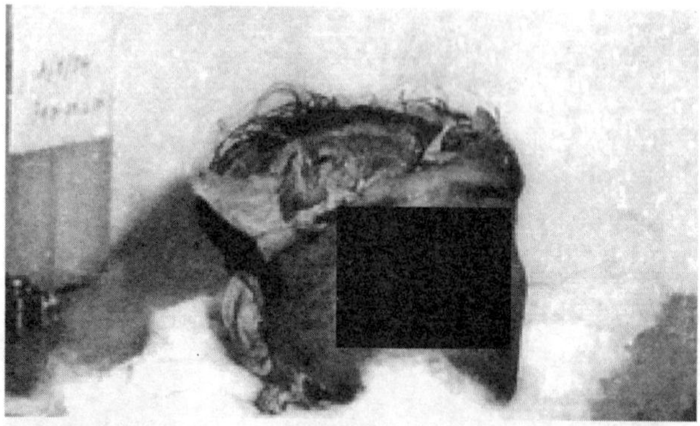

Figure 10.5: Slash/cut on uppermost part (vault) of head

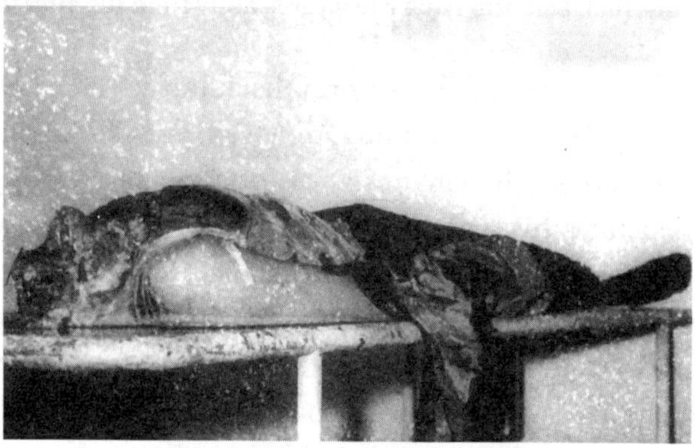

Figure 10.6: Body with intact right arm

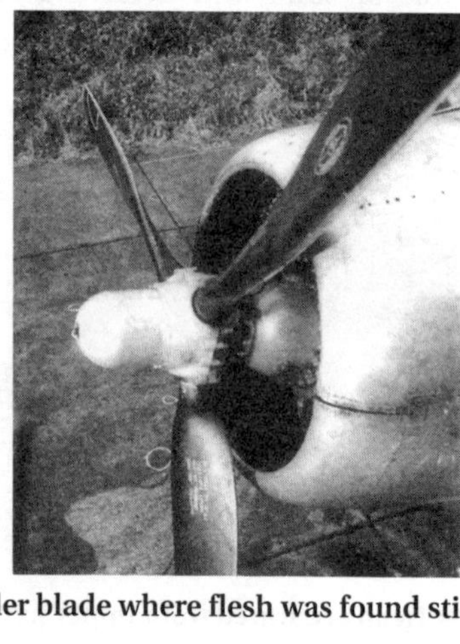

Figure 10.7: Propeller blade where flesh was found sticking (now scraped)

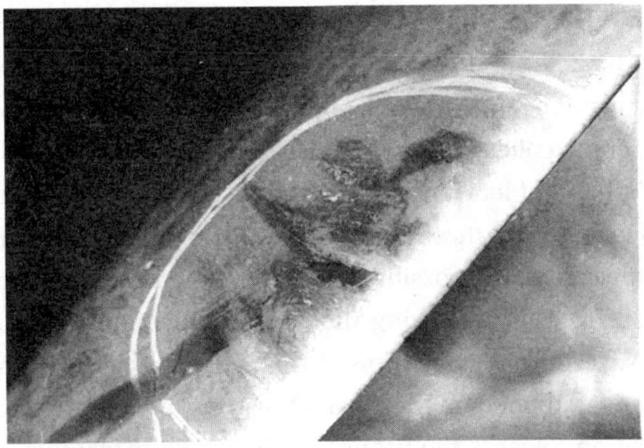

Figure 10.8: Propeller blade where tuft of hair and some flesh was sticking now removed for test)

Reconstruction of the sequence of accident posed the following questions:

(a) The pilot was a right-handed person. It is unlikely that he would hold a torchlight in his left hand and point it towards the engines. If so, how did the left arm separate from the torso?

(b) How do we explain the injury to the top of the head? If the arm and head were severed due to propeller blades, this injury had to be explained vis-à-vis the sequence of events.

With the help of an aviation medicine specialist, a thorough examination of propeller blades was made. A tuft of hair (akin to the scalp of the deceased) was found sticking to the leading edge of one blade, and some flesh and blood were noticed on the following blade. Taking into consideration the direction of rotation of blades and careful examination of their leading and trailing edges, it was suggested that the top of the head was hit first by the rotating blade and the arm and head were severed later. A full-scale dummy was used to reconstruct the sequence of events. It was found that such injuries are most unlikely if the pilot walks straight into the propeller blades. The direction and plane of injury at the vertex of the head by the rotating propeller blades was possible only if the pilot had more or less "dived" into the blades rather than "walked" into them. It was not possible to account for this "diving" action.

Examination of the flying clothing and other associated articles was undertaken. It was found that one of the flying boots of this pilot had a loose shoestring dangling from one of the shoe-eyes, as if it had been pulled out forcibly. Some colleagues of the deceased later told us "off the record" that he had a habit of leaving the shoestrings loose and was often advised against it. However, as these items were not examined on the spot by concerned specialists, the possibility that the morgue attendant had pulled at the shoestring while removing the shoes from the body could not be precluded. Nevertheless, we surmised that the pilot, while in front of the propeller blades, stepped on the loose shoestring and stumbled forward in a diving position towards the propellers. First, the presenting part of the head was slashed and then, as the body hurled further, other blades severed the arm and head. This explanation, however, remained confined to a list of "possibilities". The lessons learnt from this investigation were:

(a) Cooperation and liaison between pathologist and aviation medicine specialist/flight surgeon yields useful results.
(b) An expeditious arrival of pathologist at the scene of accident is of immense value as vital evidence and useful clues can be observed on the spot and recorded, before getting vitiated.

Investigation 3

A twin-seat training aircraft flown by an instructor and pupil pilot crashed in a field, possibly resulting from engine failure. Investigation revealed extensive damage to the aircraft and cockpit as a result of the massive forward deceleration. Both pilots were found dead by villagers who were working in the nearby fields. They removed the bodies of pilots from the wreckage. The rescue team reached the spot within a few hours and deposited the bodies in hospital mortuary.

I was requisitioned next day to perform the autopsies. Significant features, common to both fatalities, were:

(a) Both bodies showed 'caving in' of faces, especially in the frontal and maxillary areas.
(b) There were corresponding haemorrhages in the sinuses and also in the base and frontal lobes of the brain.

(c) The frontal and maxillary bones were fractured.

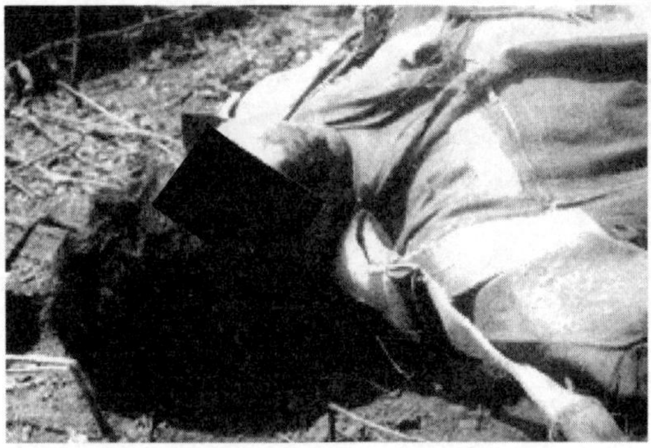

Figure 10.9: Body of pupil pilot showing 'caving in' of the face

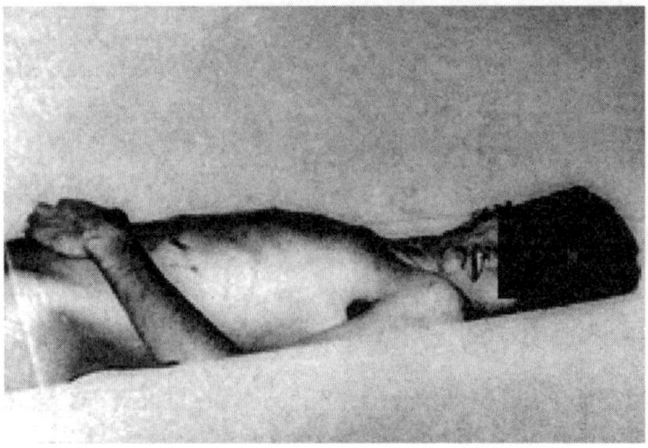

Figure 10.10: Body of pupil pilot, showing damage to face

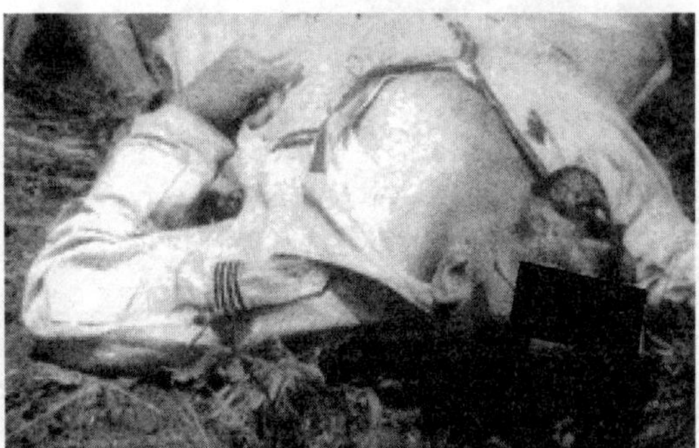

Figure 10.11: Body of instructor showing extensive injury to the face

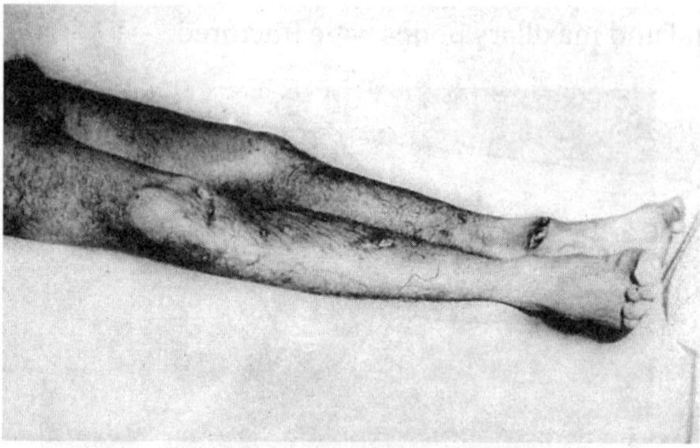

Figure 10.12: Relatively intact lower extremities (pupil pilot)

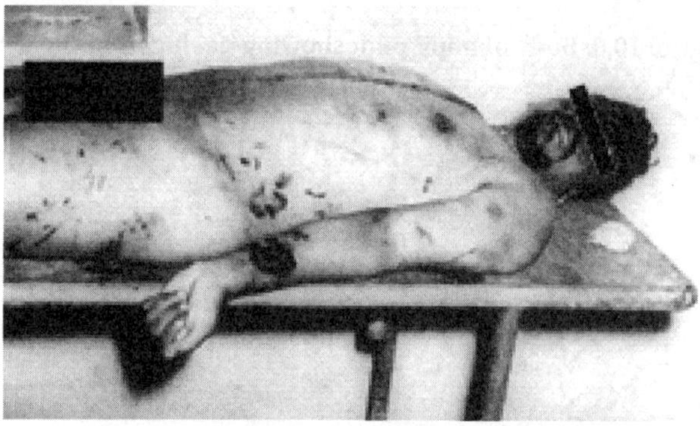

Figure 10.13: Relatively intact body of instructor (except facial injuries)

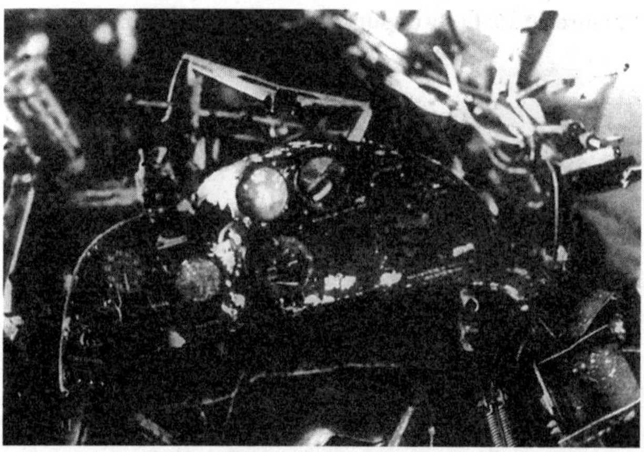

Figure 10.14: Extensively damaged cockpit

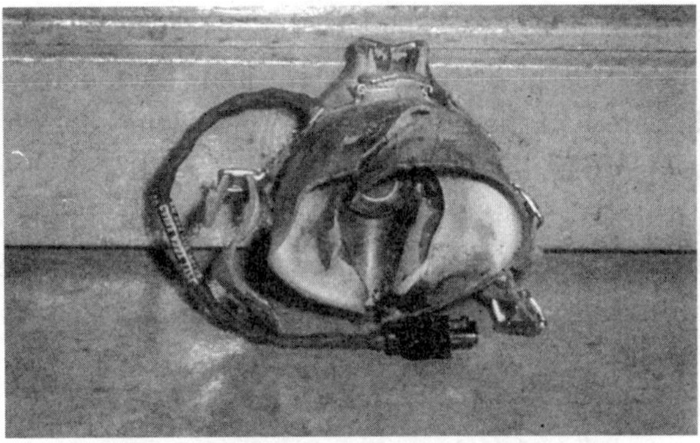

Figure 10.15: Bleeding in mask (instructor)

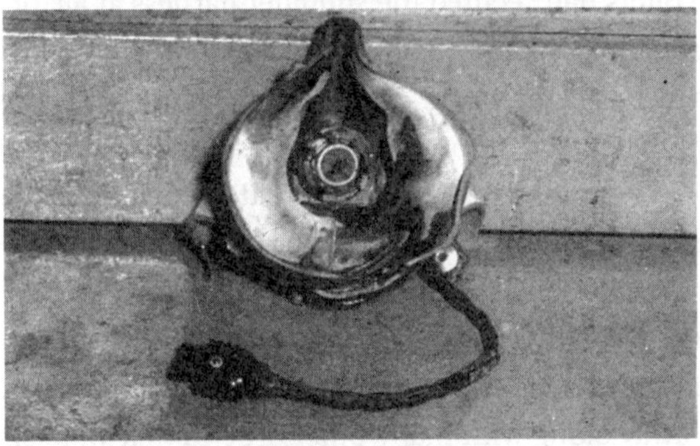

Figure 10.16: Bleeding in mask (pupil pilot)

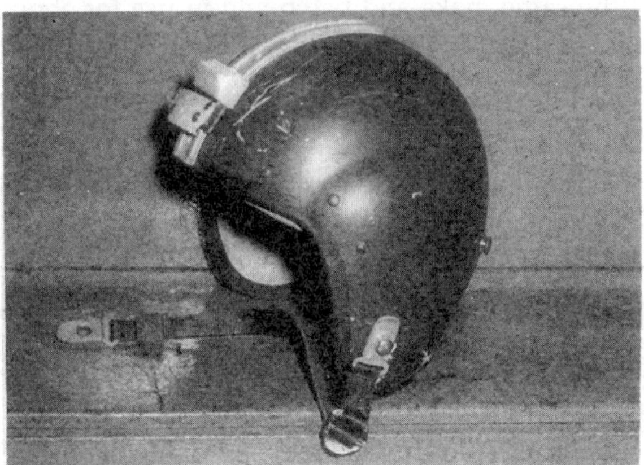

Figure 10.17: Scratches on helmet of instructor (note trailing edge of scratch)

The cause of death was attributed to fractures of bones at the base of the skull and face along with contusion and haemorrhages in the corresponding areas of the brain. Surprisingly, there were no significant injuries anywhere else in the bodies of either pilot, except for some lacerations in the extremities. Head injuries were obviously due to the heads dashing against the instrument panel, due to abrupt deceleration. Scratches in the helmet (which was otherwise intact), and blood on the instrument panel of the aircraft corroborated this.

In case of abrupt forward deceleration, the shoulder harness is meant to restrain the upper part of the body. The Court of Inquiry tried to determine whether the pilots had secured the shoulder harness at all, or whether the harnesses had broken and allowed the head to move forward. If the harnesses had taken the brunt of the deceleration force, however, there should have been corresponding marks/contusions in the region of shoulders. A re-examination of the bodies did not reveal any such evidence. It, therefore, appeared that either the pilots had not secured the harnesses or that the harnesses had snapped suddenly due to abrupt force.

A thorough search for shoulder harnesses was made in vain. (Most probably, village urchins, who had gathered there in large numbers, had taken them away along with many other articles that were strewn among the wreckage). Therefore, stress tests were performed on shoulder harnesses of the same make and batch and in use for about same time. Many of these harnesses did not conform to established standards, breaking when subjected to 'g'-forces of much lesser intensity than what was claimed in the specifications.

Therefore, although evidence regarding the snapping of the shoulder harnesses could not be directly confirmed, it brought into focus the definition of Aviation an Accident Pathology described by Mason,[1] who emphasised that findings at autopsy must be correlated with structural damage to aircraft and use/abuse of safety equipment so that a complete picture of accident may be formed. It was also realised that if an aviation pathologist was brought to the accident site immediately, he could have thought of this possibility and helped in the retrieval of shoulder harnesses.

Investigation 4

A passenger airliner took off from a coastal airport in India around midnight on an international flight. Almost immediately after take-off, it was reported to have crashed over the sea. Rescue teams arrived promptly. There were no survivors, and the bodies that were recovered from the sea over the next few days were in various stages of decomposition.

Eyewitnesses who had seen the aircraft going down gave conflicting evidence. Some described it as "flat ditching" whereas others were sure that it was a "nose-dive". Technical teams were engaged in retrieval of the engine and the flight information data recorder. I was summoned for this investigation and arrived on the same day. Bodies that were recovered from the sea were being preserved in the mortuary of a local medical college and had to be displayed in the day-time to permit identification by relatives and friends. As complete air conditioning was not possible in such a big hall, prompt identification and disposal of bodies was the main aim of the coroner.

When I requested the responsible medico-legal authorities to order autopsies, I was met with stiff resistance. In their view, the cause of death was quite apparent and the cause of the accident did not fall within their purview. It took quite some time to convince them to agree to "partial autopsies". Consequently, all bodies were X-rayed and subjected to limited autopsies. Salient features of this investigation were:

(a) All bodies were 'transected' at the level of the waist, with the lower portion missing in most cases.

(b) Heads were smashed, flattened and sometimes missing. (Figure 10.18 to Figure 10.22)

(c) X-rays of the torso showed relatively intact inter-vertebral spaces of spine but transection at various levels near the waist. There was evidence of injuries due to force acting in the transverse direction of spine and not vertical. There was no telescoping of the vertebrae (Figure 10.23 to Figure 10.25).

(d) Findings were similar in the bodies of passengers and those of air-hostesses/stewards who were identified by their uniforms/dresses.

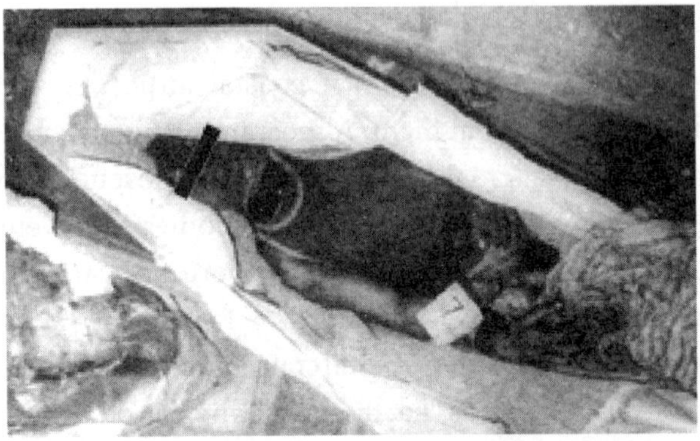

Figure 10.18: Body transected at waist with damage to head

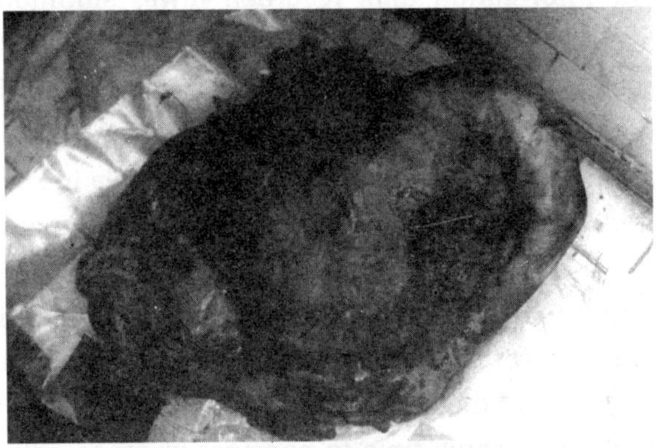

Figure 10.19: Body transected at waist with head missing

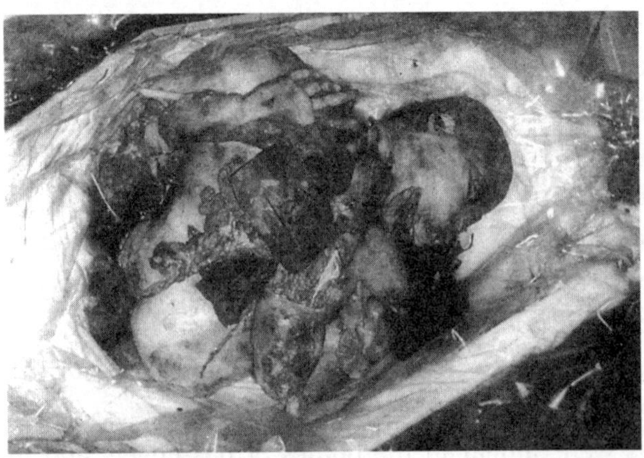

Figure 10.20: Body transected at waist with injured front of the face

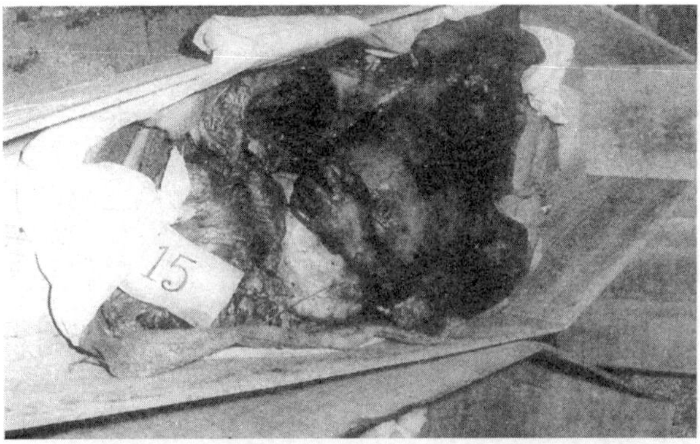

Figure 10.21: Transected body with head missing

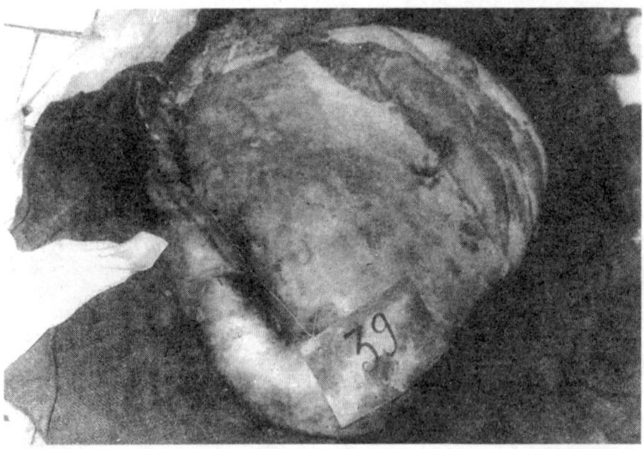

Figure 10.22: Transected body with head & neck missing

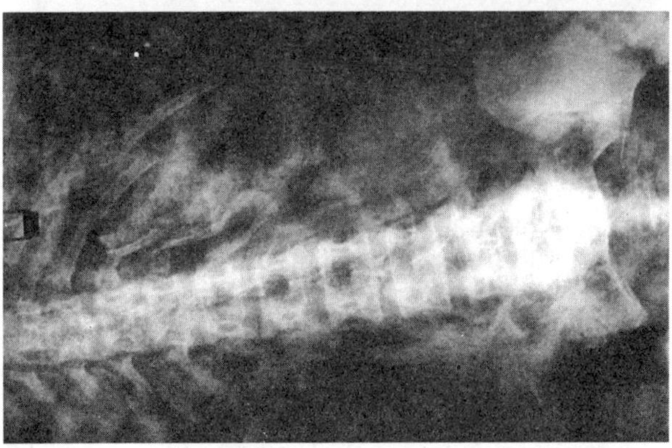

Figure 10.23: Spine showing relatively intact inter-vertebral spaces

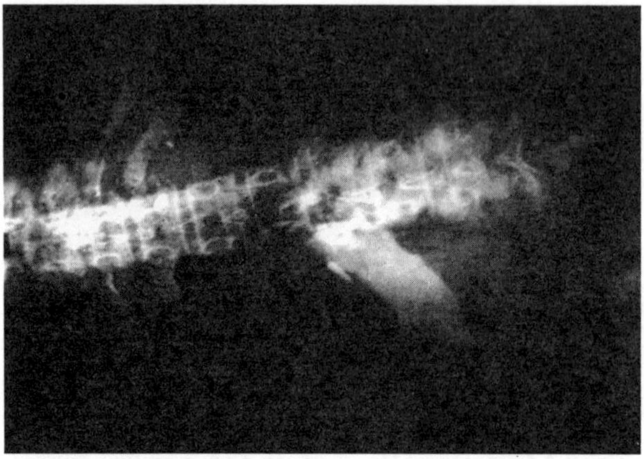

Figure 10.24: Spine shows damage due to transversally acting force

No telescoping of vertebrae to indicate vertical force acting in long-axis of spine.

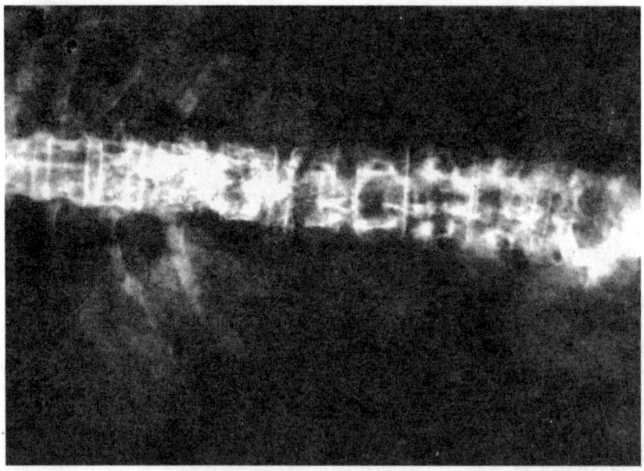

Figure 10.25: Findings show damage due to force acting in transverse direction and not in vertical, as inter-vertebral spaces are relatively intact

The above findings helped to determine the intensity and direction of the force that the passengers sustained. This force was clearly in the transverse axis of the bodies. As the lap-belts were secured during take-off, the bodies were transected at the waist level. "Bashing up" and flattening of the heads could be due to impact against the back of the seats in front.

In a passenger aircraft, airhostesses/stewards sit on their assigned seats-and fasten seat belts on take-off, landing and whenever there is an impending emergent situation. In this case, the aircraft had just taken off and, therefore, it was logical to assume that all occupants were sitting with their seat belts fastened. As crash forces operated in the transverse axis of bodies, it can be deduced that this was possible only when aircraft went into a dive and impacted on the surface of sea at almost a right angle (nosedive). This fact was later corroborated by technical evidence. Moreover, my report helped investigating authorities to rule out toxicological factors and injuries that could have been caused by explosives.

Investigation 5

A dual jet trainer aircraft having side-by-side seats flew with instructor and pupil pilot on a training exercise. Both pilots had type Q masks and Mk-17F regulators at normal setting. Within a few minutes of take-off, the control tower lost contact with the aircraft. It was found that aircraft had crashed in a field approximately 15 minutes after take-off.

A rescue team found the wreckage very soon. The aircraft was extensively damaged due to crash impact and fire. The body of the instructor was in the wreckage and completely charred. The pupil's body was lying close to the ejection seat and parachute pack, away from the wreckage. The ejection seat was apparently detached from the aircraft due to the impact of the crash as its firing mechanism was not initiated.

The pupil pilot's flying overalls were damaged and torn, but unburnt. The body showed no evidence of burns but there were extensive injuries. Part of the head and face was missing, the larynx was fractured and the thoracic cage was crushed. The tracheal mucosa was intensely congested and contained soot particles in its lower part at the bifurcation of trachea. The diaphragm, heart and abdominal viscera were ruptured, lacerated and crushed.

The cause of death, as ascertained by a clinical pathologist, was "multiple unsurvivable injuries". However, a senior aviation pathologist who was made available later, pointed out the cherry-pink colour of tissues, organs and blood, which was characteristic of carboxy-haemoglobin.

Toxicological investigations were carried out on blood samples, which showed absence of alcohol but 42 per cent concentration of carboxy-haemoglobin.

Although the body of this flyer did not show any evidence of burns, the cherry-red colour of his blood/tissues and soot particles in the lower respiratory tract suggested that he had inhaled smoke/fire when alive. As the body was found more than 15 feet away from the wreckage and had extensive injuries, the possibility of inhaling smoke or fire from the burning wreckage was virtually ruled out. Though he was a moderate smoker, such high levels of carboxy-haemoglobin could not have been caused due to cigarette smoking. It was later established that there was an in-flight fire. The Mk 17F Regulator gives air up to an altitude of only 8,000 feet through the oxygen mask at a "normal setting". In such instances, if cockpit air is contaminated with smoke or fire fumes, the same will be inhaled by the pilot. The cause of accident was therefore established as pilot incapacitation (irrespective of who was in control) that resulted from carbon monoxide intoxication due to in-flight inhalation of smoke/fire fumes.[121]

The five aforementioned instances are narrated with the sole intention of emphasising the importance of aviation accident pathology in relation to conventional medico-legal investigations. This subject is now recommended for inclusion in the syllabus for postgraduate training in pathology. As repeatedly mentioned, nothing but involvement, logical thinking and group approach delivers the results. The more one knows, the more one sees!

PART 2: APPLIED TOXICOLOGY

CHAPTER 1

TOXIC HAZARDS IN AIRCRAFT

As early as 1963, Colonel Domanski of the Armed Forces Institute of Pathology, Washington stated that a comprehensive toxicological service is essential to the medical investigation of aircraft accidents. Along with Goldbaum, he worked out a procedure for making a rapid analysis of therapeutic quantities of some commonly used drugs in the biological material. In 1967, a section of Aviation Toxicology was formed at the home office of the Central Research Establishment at Aldermaston, England, to deal with problems associated with this type of analysis. In the years to come, aviation toxicology departments were established at aviation pathology establishments in many countries. In India, a department of aviation toxicology was added to the already existing Aviation Pathology Department in 1971, at the Institute of Aviation Medicine, Bangalore.

The main aim of toxicological investigation in fatal aircraft accidents is the detection of toxic substances in biological samples of occupants and an understanding of their implications for reconstructing the accident. This discipline essentially entails the detection of substances that may have had a direct effect on the pilot prior to the accident and the determination of toxic substances like carbon monoxide and lactic acid on selected passengers and aircrew. This can provide evidence of fire or hypoxia prior to the crash. The detection of carbon monoxide, engineering fluids, aviation fuels and a wide range of medicaments is therefore required.[117,118,119,120] This objective is discussed in the following paragraphs.

During the operation of an aircraft, the pilot has two environments, each of which may be affected by toxic elements. The *external* environment may be hypoxic or contaminated by injurious elements from aviation fuels, hydraulic fluids or chemicals from various aircraft systems. This environment can be vitiated by carbon monoxide that might come from a leak of exhaust fumes or in-flight fire. Toxic elements from the environment also include carbon dioxide, oxides of nitrogen, hydrogen cyanide, sulphur dioxide, halogens and hydrocarbons.

On the other hand, the *internal* environment is inside the pilot's body itself, and may contain toxic substances such as carbon monoxide due to smoking, alcohol due to drinking, lactic acid due to hypoxia, and drugs due to deliberate medication. Commonly used drugs are non-steroid anti-inflammatory medicines, tranquillisers, hypnotics, stimulants, decongestants and anti-pyretics.

These toxic substances may arise in personal compartments of an aircraft from various aircraft systems such as exhaust gases, fire extinguishers etc. They may also be generated by excessive heat (e.g. overheating of electrical equipment), by fire that acts on materials present in the aircraft or by the firing of combat weapons from within the personnel compartment. When this happens, individuals who are present are exposed to toxic agents until such substances become dissipated or personnel are evacuated after landing.

Although extreme care is exercised during the designing of aircraft, unusual circumstances can allow toxic gases and vapours to permeate the cockpit or passenger compartment. Consequently, dangerous physiological effects, due to a combination of toxicity, concentration and prolonged exposure, are liable to occur. Unlike the toxic exposure in ground maintenance conditions, where the ground crew may be exposed on a regular basis, exposures to toxic chemicals during flight are usually of short duration and high concentration. The toxic consequences are, therefore, usually acute.

The primary toxic hazard in airborne operations is inhalation, which makes it difficult to determine the exact amount of toxic substance actually inhaled, as the effective dosage of the toxic agent is also influenced by several factors such as ambient temperature, humidity, physical activity, hyperventilation and altitude. All these factors, which are commonly present in airborne activities in varying degrees, make it very difficult to accurately determine the intensity of toxic exposure. A further complication with inhalation exposure is the simultaneous exposure to more than one contaminant. There are very few circumstances in which exposure can clearly be attributed to only one toxic material.

Sources of Toxic Hazard in Aircraft during Normal Flight

Contamination of the external environment (inside the aircraft) may result from exhaust gases, hydraulic fluids, fuels, lubricants, refrigeration and de-icing fluids, fire extinguishers, thermal decomposition products from electrical insulations, breathing oxygen system and the cargo. A consideration of combustible products is important in this context. All combustible material containing carbon may produce carbon dioxide and carbon monoxide: Celluloid, polyurethane or turbine engine starting fuels are sources of nitrogen oxides; sulphur dioxide originates from rubber and hydrogen cyanide from plastics that contain nitrogen; halogen acids are produced by poly-vinyl chlorides and fire retardants, and oils and hydraulic fluids are sources of aldehydes.

These source materials are associated with various aircraft systems, electric insulation, cabin structure, seats and coverings. As implied by the above list, the potential toxic effect of exposure to fire products is very complex. However, many of these products irritate the eyes and mucous membranes at concentrations below those that cause impairment through intoxication. For the operating crew, appropriate protection can be provided in the form of oxygen mask assemblies. Adequate protection for passengers is more difficult. However, there are currently attempts to provide plastic hoods, which give temporary protection to passengers in the event of a fire.

Exhaust gases

In piston engine aircraft, the incomplete combustion of fuel produces carbon dioxide, methane and hydrogen. If combustion becomes more complete (as evidenced by a low fuel to air ratio), the carbon dioxide in exhaust gases increases and the carbon monoxide percentage is low. On the other hand, if the exhaust gas becomes rich, carbon monoxide increases. In jet engines, exhaust gases contain mostly carbon dioxide, and so the probability of carbon monoxide is low. However, sulphur dioxide and aldehydes may be present in the exhaust gases in sufficient quantities to produce irritation of the eyes and respiratory tract.

When new aircraft are introduced, rigid control is exercised to ensure that exhaust gases do not enter the cockpit or passenger compartment. As a result of wear and tear, however, or subsequent structural modifications, some amount of exhaust gas may still find its way inside the aircraft. Regular toxicological assessment to check the environment is necessary to avoid mishaps that result from such contamination.

Carbon monoxide

As we have already observed, the only substance of toxicological significance in exhaust gases is carbon monoxide, to which individuals during flight are exposed as a result of inhalation, besides cigarette smoking or aircraft fires. Single-engine aircraft, with the engine located in front of cockpit produce greater contamination than aircraft with multi-lateral engines.

Carbon monoxide should be suspected when fumes suggestive of heater or exhaust sources are noted. This gas is invariably associated with in-flight fire. In several instances, failures in the exhaust system have been responsible for the seepage of carbon monoxide into the cockpit. The failure was sometimes due to a crack in the exhaust stacks from excessive vibrations. In other cases, the gas entered the cockpit through worn-out packing around the collector rings. In aircraft equipped with exhaust heaters, contamination has resulted from wear and tear of intensifier tube assembly.

Because carbon monoxide is odourless, it is very difficult to detect. It is therefore necessary to use one of the various carbon monoxide detectors available to record its presence.

In high-performance military aircraft, where demand oxygen regulators are used, the danger of carbon monoxide decreases with increasing altitudes over 10,000 feet. Above 30,000 feet, where the demand system furnishes 100 per cent oxygen, the action of carbon monoxide is completely prevented. Therefore, when flying personnel suspect the presence of carbon monoxide in the aircraft because of either an odour of exhaust gas or untoward symptoms (headache, nausea, dizziness or dimming of vision), they turn off the exhaust heaters in use and switch on 100 per cent oxygen. By so doing, protection against carbon monoxide intoxication is ensured.

Hydraulic fluids

Hydraulic fluids are usually castor oil based. However, new synthetic types have also been introduced. A quantity of 20 to 50 gallons is usually present in the system, which is under high pressure. A leak in the hydraulic pipe may produce a fine spray in the personnel compartment and compounds like castor oil and aldehydes are inhaled to cause irritation of eyes, violent cough and even vertigo. Synthetic-based hydraulic fluids may enter the body even through the skin.

Fuels and Lubricants

Aircrew and passengers may be exposed to the adverse effects of aircraft engine fuels. In the case of aircrew, this can cause a performance decrement. Thus, an aviation pathologist should be conversant with broad facts about these fuels. Needless to say, these fuels vary greatly in composition and changes are made from time to time. However, we can broadly classify them into "Aviation Gasoline" (for piston-engine aircraft) and "Jet Fuels" (for jet engines). Piston-engine aircraft fuel contains various hydrocarbons along with small amounts of aniline, toluene, xylene and xylidine. A small quantity of tetra-ethyl-lead is added to prevent knocking. Some fuels, however, do not contain any lead. Jet fuels contain paraffin, similar to kerosene and aromatics. Some are mixtures of fuel oil, gasoline and kerosene along with aromatics. One variety is a narrow distillate with kerosene and aromatics.

The aviation gasoline used in piston-engine aircraft contains hydrocarbons which, if inhaled, produce nausea, headache, and giddiness. It can eventually cause intoxication and loss of consciousness if inhaled in high concentration. Aircrew and ground staff can be exposed even on the tarmac if there is a fuel spill. The smell of this gasoline is a warning sign. In low concentrations, however, it can go undetected and inadvertent inhalation can produce excitability and poor judgment.

Thermal decomposition products of electric equipment

These thermal decomposition products often contain plastic insulating materials around the wires. Heat leads these materials (especially those with phenolic resins) to liberate carbon monoxide and cyanide gases. Different types of toxic products are produced, depending upon the temperature. Teflon is the most heat resistant but is not totally so, as it is known to produce "metal fume fever". Overheating of electrical equipment and burning produce colourless gases or fumes, which can sometimes go undetected.

Fire Extinguishants

Fire extinguishants differ, depending on the material that is burning. For papers and cotton material, water and halogenated hydrocarbons may be sufficient. When inflammable substances are burning, carbon dioxide is used to cover and envelope the fire. Carbon dioxide is also used for dousing burning electrical equipment as it is a nonconductor of electricity. These substances, particularly carbon dioxide and halogenated hydrocarbons, produce respiratory distress. Carbon tetrachloride produces a narcotic effect, vomiting and liver damage.

Miscellaneous

The other substances quoted earlier are not of much significance. De-icing fluids were traditionally used to lower the freezing point of water and to prevent ice formation on propellers, windshields and carburetors. They contain some alcohols along with water and propylene/ethylene glycol. With the change to electrically-operated devices, their use is now limited. Similarly, the use of coolants and refrigerants is also limited these days. In aviation, oxygen is used in gaseous as well as liquid form. In-flight breathing of oxygen in transport flying is now rare due to cabin pressurisation but is still in vogue in military flying. In concentrations of less than 50 per cent and at standard atmospheric pressure, oxygen has no toxicity even if breathed for a long time.

CHAPTER 2

CARBON MONOXIDE AND AVIATION

Although discovered by Priestley in 1799, one or another form of carbon monoxide (CO) has been known since ancient times. It is reported to have been used by the Greeks and Romans as a means of executing criminals and committing suicide. In 1842, Leblanc attributed many accidents to a gas produced by burning coal. In 1856, Claude Bernard described its ill effects on the human body due to formation of carboxy-haemoglobin (COHb). In 1895, Haldane and Mosso worked extensively on this subject and explained how this mechanism caused "asphyxia". Nicloux, in 1903, sounded a hopeful note to state that the effects of CO are reversible as the gas dissociates itself from haemoglobin by exposure to oxygen.

Almost all flames and combustion devices emit carbon monoxide. It is present in the exhausts of internal combustion engines, illuminating and heating gases and is held responsible for about 3,500 accidental or suicidal deaths per year in the US. In aviation, cockpit contamination with carbon monoxide may incapacitate the pilot with disastrous results, particularly at high altitudes. Toxic effects of this gas are due to hypoxia. The affinity of the haemoglobin molecule for CO is about 250 times greater than it is for oxygen. Consequently, it competes with oxygen and combines with haemoglobin even if its concentration is very low (0.02–0.04 per cent). Regarded as one of the chief toxicological villains, CO is known to have caused many aircraft accidents. In India, one such accident was recorded in a trainer aircraft in 1977, as reported by Kapur et al.[121] Blackmore[122] and Mason[1] have described several such accidents in details. Dille and Linder[123] have also found it to be responsible for a significant number of aircraft accidents.

Physical and Chemical Properties

Carbon monoxide, which is usually produced by incomplete combustion of carbonaceous material, is a colourless, odourless, tasteless and non-irritating gas. It, therefore, can be inhaled unknowingly. It burns in air with a blue flame to produce carbon dioxide (CO_2). With a molecular weight of 28.01, vapour density 14, water solubility 3 per cent, its density of 0.076 is approximately that of air, which makes it highly diffusible.

As it acts as a reducing agent, oxides of iron or copper can be reduced to form iron and copper, a property which is used in tests to detect its presence. In the presence of certain catalysts such as zinc or chromium oxides, a mixture of CO and hydrogen under pressure of 200–300 atmospheres can produce methanol.

Sources of Carbon Monoxide in Aviation

Exhaust fumes from a reciprocating engine may contain 5–15 per cent CO. This percentage is 8.75 at take-off and 3.03 while cruising. However, fire can increase the concentrations to dangerous levels. Single-engine aircraft, with motors in front of the fuselage are more vulnerable to contamination than are aircraft with multiple-lateral engines. In fixed-wing aircraft, CO may enter the cockpit through a leak from the combustion system. It can also be generated by excessive heat, e.g. overheating of electric and fire equipment.

Failure of the exhaust system in the form of cracks in the exhaust stack, due to excessive vibrations, has been responsible for several instances of CO-seepage in the cockpit. The gas can sometimes enter through worn-out packing around collector rings. In aircraft that are fitted with exhaust heaters, contamination has resulted from a worn-out intensifier tube assembly. In helicopters, carbon monoxide can enter the cabin because of rotor action during hovering as well as coming from the combustion system.

Permitted Concentration of CO

A concentration of 0.005 per cent is permitted in passenger aircraft in the USA. Variable concentration has been allowed by the American Standard

Association, depending upon the duration of exposure. For instance, exposure to 0.01 per cent of CO for a period not exceeding 8 hours a day, and 0.04 per cent for a period not exceeding one hour a day, are the upper limits. With these exposures, carboxyhaemoglobin formed in the blood is 7 per cent, which is the concentration usually encountered in the blood of heavy smokers.

Concentration of CO in Aviation

With advancement in technology, aircrew duties are becoming more and more demanding. Combat flying necessitates split-second decisions based upon the inputs from various complex electronic gadgets, and the performance capability of aircrew with respect to critical tasks can often be marginal. In such cases, even a minor degree of bodily impairment due to CO can greatly increase the possibility of pilot error. Exceeding the permissible concentrations noted earlier may not only affect ground personnel but also influence the performance of the aircrew. It has been demonstrated experimentally that impairment of vision occurs even at concentrations below the allowable limits.

Duration of Exposure

Exposure to CO is usually of short duration, depending on flying time. In fighter aircraft, it may even be less than one or two hours. The relation between the concentration of CO in inhaled air and the danger resulting from exposure to it is as follows:

Percentage of CO	**Degree of danger in relation to exposure time**
Less than 0.04	Allowable for several hours
0.04–0.05	No appreciable effect in one hour
0.06–0.07	Just appreciable effect after 1 hour
0.1–0.12	Unpleasant but not dangerous after 1 hour
0.15–0.2	Dangerous in 1 hour
0.4 and above	Fatal in less than 1 hour

The above values are based on exposure to constant concentrations. In practice, concentrations vary over time. One must take into account the fact that the period of allowable exposure to a given concentration is decreased as a result of prior exposures. This concern becomes important, for example, when a flyer is a heavy smoker and has smoked before flying (resulting in a baseline level of CO as 7–8 per cent). Thus, the permissible period and permissible concentrations have to be interpreted cautiously.

Effects of High Altitudes

At high altitudes oxygen partial pressure is lower and CO thus combines with a greater amount of haemoglobin. Consequently, there is an increase in CO toxicity and impairment of performance. For example, if an individual has 8 per cent carboxyhaemoglobin in his blood at an altitude of 4,000 feet, he will be affected at 11,000 feet of altitude. Some workers have reported that 3 per cent carboxyhaemoglobin at 15,000 feet produces an effect equal to that of 20 per cent carboxyhaemoglobin at sea level. The total effect is compounded due to the fact that the supply of oxygen to tissues is already inadequate at high altitudes and the oxygen-carrying capacity of the blood is low due to exposure to CO. Blood loss at high altitudes can therefore produce disastrous effects.

Other Factors influencing CO Toxicity

Factors in addition to the concentration of inhaled gas and exposure time come into apply when assessing CO toxicity. These include:

(a) Rate of lung-ventilation
(b) Blood volume (size of individual)
(c) Haemoglobin concentration
(d) Rate of elimination
(e) Susceptibility of individual

Some of the above deserve serious consideration. The rate of ventilation, for example, influences the rate of uptake of CO, as this gas, when inhaled, continues to combine with haemoglobin and gradually carboxyhaemoglobin concentration builds up. The expected increase in concentration of COHb also depends upon the physical work involved. A formula is given below:

increase in % of COHb = K X % of CO X minutes of exposure., when

K = 3 for rest (ventilation rate 6 litres/mt, pulse 70/mt)

= 5 for light activity (ventilation @9 ltr/mt, pulse 80/mt)

= 8 for moderate activity (ventilation @18 ltr/mt, pulse 110/mt)

= 11 for heavy work (ventilation @30 ltr/mt, pulse 135/mt)

Piloting an aircraft amounts to "light work" and thus a concentration of COHb of 7 per cent should not be exceeded. Hence, one can calculate the time required to reach this level while breathing different concentrations of CO:

Concentration of CO (%)	Minutes to reach 7% COHb level
0.02	88
0.03	29
0.05	18
0.1	9
0.2	4

The aforementioned equation needs to be corrected for high altitudes, depending upon partial pressure of CO in the trachea and lungs at specific altitudes and also for increased ventilation.

The rate of elimination of CO is slower compared to its intake. COHb declines by about 50 per cent in one to three hours. Its elimination can be speeded up by increasing lung ventilation and oxygen partial pressure.

The increase in COHb concentration in the blood is not uniform. The rate of increase is initially rapid but then gradually declines, reaching equilibrium. The time-courses of COHb concentration in the blood on exposure to breathing CO at 0.01 per cent, 0.05 per cent and 0.1 per cent in air, at rest and light work are shown Figure 2.1.

In high-performance aircraft, where demand oxygen regulators are used, the danger of CO poisoning decreases with increasing altitude over 10,000 feet as 100 per cent oxygen is supplied by this system.

Physiopathology

Carbon monoxide in toxic concentration produces its effect by: (a) combining with the haemoglobin molecule, and (b) altering the

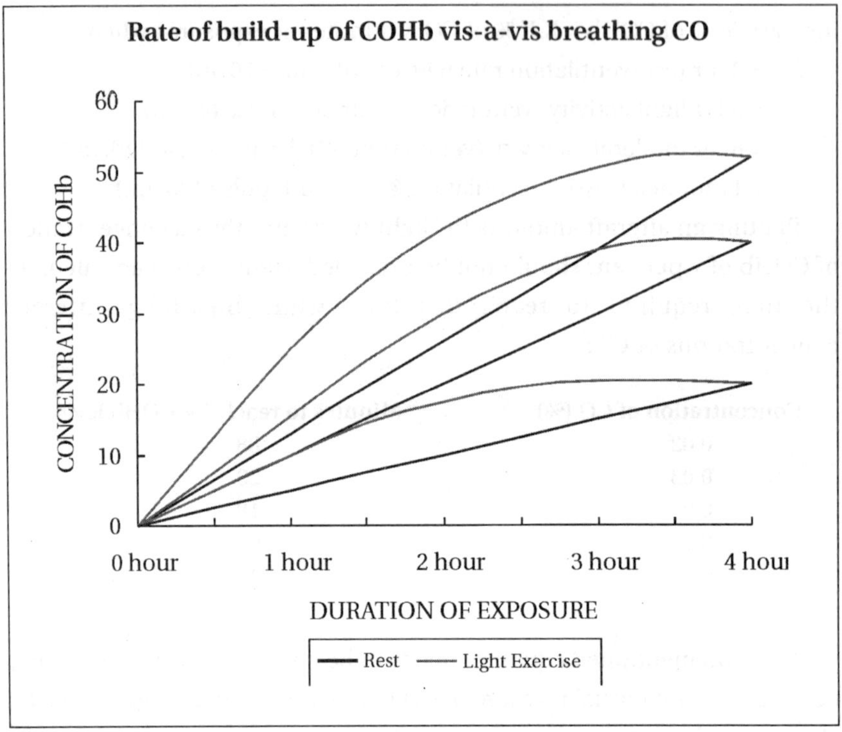

Figure 2.1

characteristics of dissociation of remaining oxy-haemoglobin by causing a "shift to left" of the oxygen-dissociation curve. Some important facets of these effects are highlighted below:

(a) **Combining with haemoglobin molecule:** CO has 250 times more affinity for haemoglobin than oxygen has. Therefore, it easily combines with haemoglobin to form carboxyhaemoglobin (COHb), thus rendering the haemoglobin incapable of combining with oxygen as well. Thus, the oxygen is displaced by CO. CO forms complexes with the oxidation-reduction system of cells, particularly affecting the enzyme cytochrome-a3- oxidase. CO, in fact, combines with the iron moiety of this enzyme, thereby preventing its utilisation and inhibiting its role as activator of molecular oxygen. Hence, it results in the blocking of cellular oxidation to cause histotoxic hypoxia.

In an atmosphere containing 10 per cent CO (e.g. the exhaust of an engine), 60 per cent of the haemoglobin will be converted into COHb within one minute. A dose of CO will be lethal if it produces 60 per cent of COHb in proportion to the total blood haemoglobin. Hence death occurs within the time that .66 of the haemoglobin has been converted. This proportion (0.66) is known as the poisoning coefficient. In normal atmospheric conditions, this coefficient is equivalent to a CO level of 1/500. The levels of poisoning coefficient in relation to clinical situations are:

Below 0.1	Usually no symptoms
0.1–0.2	Dyspnoea on exertion
0.2–0.3	Headache
0.3–0.4	Muscular adynamia, nausea, dizziness
0.4–0.5	Syncope or tendency to collapse
0.5–0.6	Convulsions
0.6–0.7	Fatal outcome if exposure is prolonged
0.8	Instantaneous death

The duration of exposure is also very important, however. Even at a coefficient of 0.2, death can occur if the subject remains too long in the vitiated atmosphere. Prolonged anoxemia produces anatomical and physiological disorders of the tissues at a cellular level. Respiratory and cardiac reactions occur, especially with hyperventilation accompanied by respiratory alkalosis — going to irreversible acidosis due to incomplete combustion and liberation of acid metabolites. The adult brain consumes about 25 per cent of the oxygen inhaled and hypoxia produces oedema of the brain and damage to white matter. Besides producing hypoxia, CO has a direct histotoxic effect on the brain. There is vascular stasis and an anoxic lesion of vascular walls produces oedema due to increased permeability. Vasostasis occurs and obstruction of small blood vessels results from either the swelling of endothelial cells or compression due to oedema of surrounding tissue.

(b) **Shift of Oxyhaemoglobin Dissociation Curve:** In the presence of COHb, the oxygen dissociation curve shifts to the left, as shown in Figure 2.2. Therefore, oxyhaemoglobin does not readily give up its oxygen to tissues. Thus, it is not only the low level of remaining oxyhaemoglobin, but also the qualitative behaviour by which it does not part with oxygen.

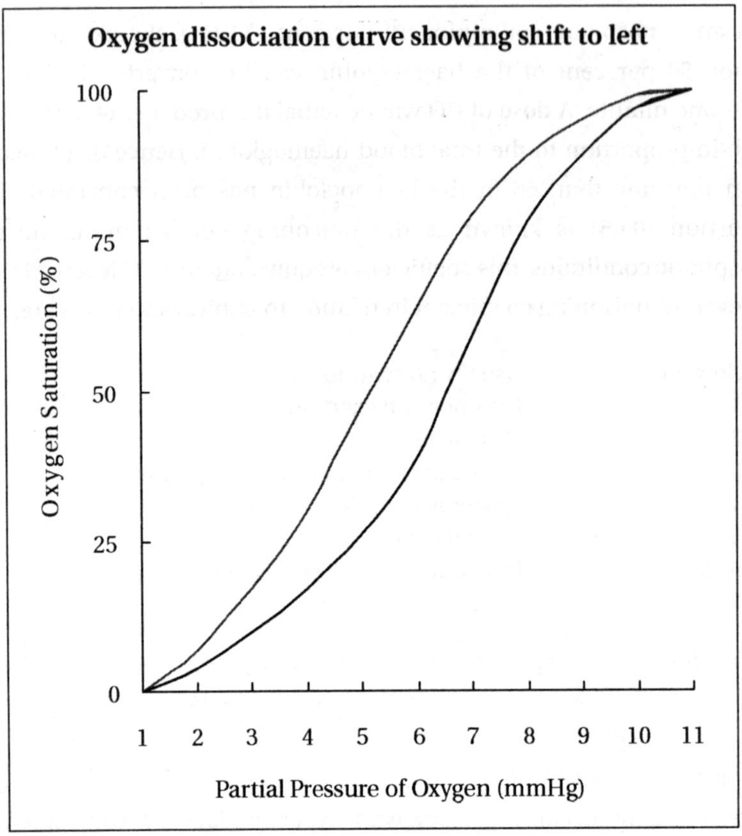

Figure 2.2

The dissociation of COHb follows the same laws as the dissociation of HbO. Thus, the COHb dissociation curve is governed by the same factors (temperature, pH and salt contents) as the HbO curve. The main difference between the two curves lies in the range of partial pressures. Haemoglobin becomes 50 per cent saturated with PO_2 at about 30 mm Hg but becomes 50 per cent saturated with CO at 0.12 mm Hg. Hence, inspiration of air containing even 0.1 per cent CO will cause symptoms of intoxication with 30 to 60 minutes. As the HbO dissociation curve is also displaced to the left in the presence of CO, this results in a marked lowering of partial pressure at which oxygen is available for tissue metabolism. Thus, despite the presence of two or three times the amount of oxygen necessary for normal tissue functions, profound anoxia develops early in CO poisoning. One individual who is anaemic might appear reasonably well even if concentration of haemoglobin has fallen by 50 per cent of normal, whereas another person whose haemoglobin is 50 per cent saturated with CO would be practically dead (Figure 2.3).

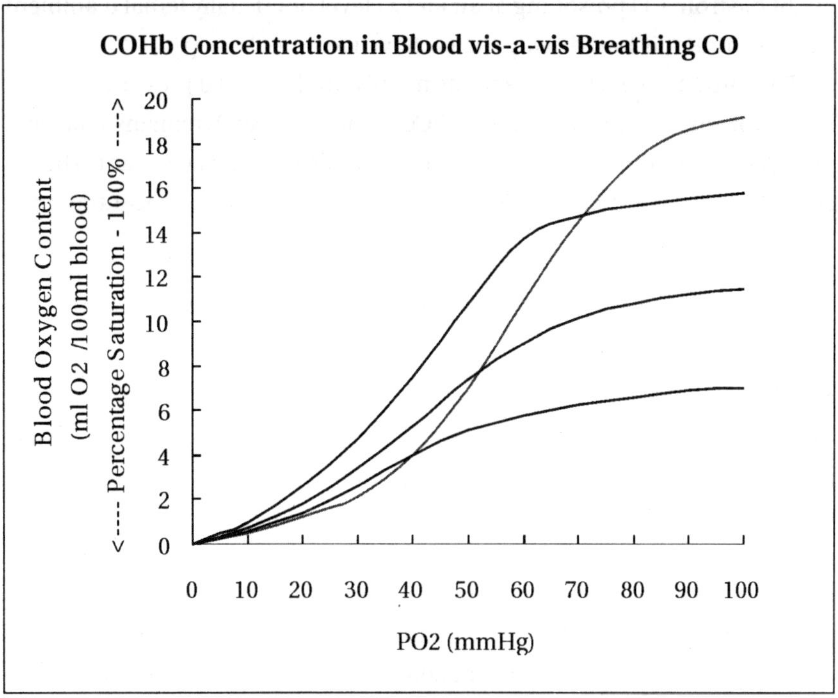

Figure 2.3

The relationship between the concentration of COHb and HbO_2 under conditions in which two gases are present in quantities sufficient to saturate the haemoglobin is given by the Haldane Equation (COHb is shown as HbCO and HbO as HbO_2):

$$\frac{[HbCO]}{[HbO_2]} = M\frac{PCO}{PO_2}$$

This equation relates the partial pressure of carbon monoxide in the air, the partial pressure of oxygen in the air and the concentrations of carboxyhaemoglobin and oxyhaemoglobin in the blood. "M" is known as

Haldane's constant and is equal to approximately 200. Carboxyhaemoglobin will be increased by increasing the partial pressure of carbon monoxide (i.e. increase in ppm CO) and/or by decreasing the partial pressure of ambient oxygen (i.e. depleting oxygen). This means that one might die from CO poisoning at an air CO level not usually lethal if ambient oxygen content is low, driving the carboxyhaemoglobin up.

The formation of HbCO depends mainly on the partial pressure of CO. It is evident that the proportion of HbCO relative to HbO_2 remains constant, provided the amount of CO in relation to O_2 also remains constant. Thus, a concentration of .01per cent CO in air results in the ratio of concentration of

$$\frac{210 \times 0.01 \times barometric\ pressure}{20.9 \times barometric\ pressure} \quad OR \quad \frac{\%\ HbCO}{\%\ HbO_2} = 0.1$$

Effects of CO Inhalation

The leading symptoms of CO intoxication are headache, weakness, vertigo, nervousness, dyspnoea, parasthesia, muscular twitching, emotional disturbances, nausea, drowsiness, cough, sweating, vomiting, precordial distress, vasomotor instability, impairment of speech, loss of hearing, hoarseness of voice and yawning. The ophthalmic manifestations after prolonged repeated exposure include a narrowing of visual fields, amblyopia, anisocornea, retinal oedema, diplopia and neuro-retinitis.

In acute poisoning, there are fewer symptoms as unconsciousness occurs quickly. The greatest individual variation in symptoms is encountered when the exposure has been less severe, more protracted and repeated.

In aviation, COHb, even at lower concentrations, can result in fatality by impairing finer judgments of all faculties and adversely affecting the altitude tolerance, visual functions and general performance. Surprisingly, however, medical and other Federal Aviation Administration bodies show no accident that has been solely attributable to COHb levels below 8 per cent.

Dille and Linder[123] analyzed the records of 2,660 fatal general aviation aircraft accidents. CO was found as a cause in 5 of them, with COHb levels from 12 per cent to 33 per cent. They concluded that impaired vision, reduced altitude tolerance and fatigue might have contributed to some of these accidents. Alcohol, altitude and CO have additive effects. The mechanism of CO toxicity has been highlighted by Goldbaum et al.[124, 125]

Tests of higher cerebral functions (e.g. the ability to sense the flickering in a rhythmically flashing light, ability to discriminate between short intervals of time and simple choice discrimination) have demonstrated deterioration in the performance of persons having even low levels of COHb. Levels as low as 5 per cent affect performance in some of these tests. Complex psychological functions involving judgment, situational decisions and corrective responses are likely to be affected by exposure to levels of CO that produce concentrations of COHb between 5 and 20 per cent. COHb in a smoker can increase up to 8 per cent and can reduce night-vision acuity, increase susceptibility to hypoxia and prolong the time for dark adaptation.

Estimation of COHb in Blood

Toxicological investigations of this nature should be conducted at a toxicological laboratory only where necessary expertise is available. Thus, only broad principles involved in the tests are mentioned below.

The biological samples required during autopsy for estimation of COHb are: (a) blood (5–10 ml) and (b) muscle tissue (100 gm). Ideally, samples should be frozen in a dark glass bottle with a layer of liquid paraffin on the top. Samples should be protected from sunlight to prevent deterioration of CO.

Before proceeding with detailed tests, some screening tests are desirable.

(a) *Naked eye examination:* Diluted blood (1 to 2 drops in 5 ml of water) shows yellowish red colour of HbO and pinkish (cherry) red colour of COHb.

(b) *The Alkali test:* Two drops of test blood sample and 2 drops of control normal blood are placed separately on a white tile. Add 2 drops of 25 per cent sodium hydroxide to each and mix. The colour of COHb remains the same as it resists alkali denaturation while the normal control sample turns brown. This test can detect COHB of only 20 per cent or more. Results should be observed within one minute.

(c) *The Takayama test:* This test can detect up to 10 per cent COHb in blood. Take 5 drops of test blood and 5 drops of normal control blood sample. Add 5 drops of fresh orange-coloured ammonium sulphide to each. Make it acidic with a few drops of acetic acid. A rose colour will develop if COHb is present. Otherwise, in a normal sample the colour will be a dirty greenish brown.

(d) *Spectroscopy:* HbO shows 2 bands in spectroscopy. By using a reducing agent like sodium dithionate, HbO is converted to Hb and two bands will be replaced by only one band, which also shifts a little to the left. If COHb is present, no such change will occur.

(e) *Differential protein precipitation:* This test is based upon the principle that HbO is almost completely precipitated at pH 5.28 by heating at 57°C for 8 minutes, while approximately 80 per cent of COHb remains in solution. After precipitation of HbO, presence of COHb can be calculated colorimetrically against a COHb standard.

(f) *Spectrophotometry:* COHb has absorption peaks at 535 nm and 570.5 nm. Out of these, the former is a bigger peak. However, HbO has absorption peaks at 576.5 nm and 544.8 nm, the former being a bigger peak than the latter.

(g) *Liberation of CO and subsequent measurement:* Whole blood is treated with a reagent to liberate CO, which is measured by chemical or other physico-chemical means. Quantification of gas is done by gas chromatography. Common gas-liberating substances are sulphuric acid, potassium ferri-cyanide and lactic acid. Final measurement is done by estimation of reduced potassium, volumetric determination or use of gas chromatography.

(h) *Gas chromatography:* This is specific and eliminates error due to the presence of compounds formed by bacterial decomposition. Quantification of CO bound to Hb in a blood haemolysate cannot be of any value unless it is related to the total concentration of Hb present. Thus, first Hb is measured by any standard method (e.g. determination of the total CO binding capacity or total iron content or the use of a spectrophotometer). COHb is measured by using a gas chromatograph fitted with the appropriate column and helium as carrier gas.

Haemolysate made earlier is transferred into a disposable plastic syringe. The de-gassing agent is transferred to this syringe by common plastic tubing attached to the syringe. After proper mixing, the air space containing CO is transferred to a 5-ml gas loop and introduced into the gas chromatograph. The recorder tracing will show separation of N, O and CO. The volume of CO is calculated and related with haemoglobin estimated earlier in the haemolysate. Determination of CO in tissues is also done on the same principle.

Some workers have warned against spurious production of CO after death during the process of decomposition. It can also be due to embalming, when a technique involving 100 per cent carboxylation is used. Pre-treatment with a reducing agent rules out this possibility. Weak embalming solutions do not increase concentration of CO. No loss of CO is reported on storage at 37°C, even for 4 hours.

(i) In addition to the tests described above, there are highly specialised procedures such as Thin Layer Chromatography and Atomic Absorption Sectrophotometry. In high-performance aircraft accidents, the fatalities are in a mutilated and fragmented state. In the absence of intact bodies, the investigations have to be performed on small amounts of blood extracted from tissues. Under such circumstances, these procedures may have to be employed.

(j) In living persons who are suspected of having been exposed to CO, COHb can be estimated by a simple screening method using a balloon, a Drager's gas analysis kit and CO detector tubes (0.001 per cent). The tube, which produces colour when exposed to exhaled gas, shows the number marked on it, which gives the percentage of CO present in the breath. This is equated with the percentage of COHb by means of a graph, which is provided with the kit.

Interpretation

Certain basic facts, summarized below, must be kept in mind when interpreting the results:

(a) COHb levels up to 5 per cent can be encountered in any individual, especially a smoker. Levels up to 8 per cent can be found in chronic smokers and, therefore, a history of smoking must be carefully elucidated.

(b) Although levels between 5 and 9 per cent may indicate possible exposure to CO while alive, such cases must be evaluated in the light of all known crash factors and circumstantial evidence.

(c) All levels above 10 per cent indicate exposure when alive, either in flight or at the time of crash. In cases of survival, high concentrations of COHb may be encountered for a period of time in the vitiated atmosphere containing CO. Common forms of exposure reported are smoking, inhalation of exhaust fumes and fire.

(d) When evaluating the circumstances of an accident, the following facts must be borne in mind:

(i) The major problem of CO exposure in aviation is insidious marginal impairment in matters of judgment, especially during an emergency. This impairment can occur at even lower levels of COHb (10–20 per cent).

ii) Hypoxia produces an additional effect. Heavy smoking, with COHb levels of 5–10 per cent, will produce hypoxia equivalent to 5,000–7,000 feet in altitude. If such an individual is exposed to a cabin altitude of 5,000–7,000 feet, his or her performance will be approximately equivalent to that at 10,000–14,000 feet.

iii) On cessation of exposure, CO will slowly be eliminated by breathing air at sea level. Elimination half-time is about 1 to 2 hours. With breathing pure oxygen at the same level, it will be from 30 to 45 minutes. These times will vary with altitude.

(e) The maximum allowed concentration of CO is 100 ppm of air (0.01 per cent volume) for not more than 8 hours of exposure a day. Piston-engine aircrews are more likely to be exposed to CO than jet-engine aircraft crew. CO is present in large quantities in the exhaust of piston-engine aircraft. When engines are placed immediately in front of cockpits or passenger compartments, the chances of contamination through slip streams are great. Single-engine aircraft with radial engines having short exhausts are even worse in this respect.

Interpretation of Marginally Elevated Levels

During toxicological investigation of fatal aircraft accidents, grossly high levels of COHb in blood samples of aircrew/passengers leave no doubt about exposure to CO. However, an interpretation of marginally elevated levels is difficult when the total flying situation is assessed with respect to accident causation. As mentioned previously, COHb levels up to 8–10 per cent are known to exist in the blood of chronic smokers. If similar levels are encountered in the blood samples of air crew fatalities, the question generally arises as to whether these levels belong to the decline phase. In other words, these levels may have been even higher and declined due to survival in a relatively CO-free atmosphere. Second, there may be deterioration in the levels subsequent to death due to factors such as time-lag, exposure to atmosphere and sunlight.

In developing countries, when fatal accidents occur in difficult terrain, it may not be possible to reach the accident site expeditiously. Even if an autopsy is performed and blood samples are collected within a few hours of the accident, the samples are usually sent to a toxicological laboratory by courier. Some deterioration in COHb values is natural during this process. Often values like 6–8 per cent are dismissed as insignificant without considering the possibility that the levels at the time of accident might have been much higher (10–15 per cent) but may have deteriorated due to storage conditions. Some researchers (Adaval and Diwan[126]) have tried to study the deterioration rate of COHb during various conditions of storage (exposure to daylight, temperatures of 4 and 37°C and atmospheric air). They found that when blood samples had been stored for 7 days, the mean deterioration was 16.2 per cent when they had been stored in dark-coloured bottles; as compared to 21.9 per cent if they had been stored in clear glass bottles. Furthermore, the deterioration was only 6.4 per cent when they were stored at 4°C as opposed to 12.4 per cent when they were stored at 37°C. Deterioration was only 6.3 per cent when the samples were stored under liquid paraffin as opposed to 10.5 per cent when the samples were left exposed to the atmosphere. Thus, storage under liquid paraffin in dark-coloured bottles at 4°C is the ideal method of preservation. If any of these conditions cannot be met, one should take into account the deterioration factors described.

These researchers also found that the decay rate of COHb after exposure to adverse conditions mentioned above was more or less of a constant nature under each condition and could be extrapolated if required. Deterioration was found to be maximum when stored in clear bottles and exposed to atmospheric conditions (sunlight, variable temperature and in equilibrium with atmospheric air) while under ideal conditions (dark amber-coloured bottles, under liquid paraffin and at temperature of 4°C), where all adverse factors are eliminated, deterioration is minimised.

It is, therefore, recommended that when marginally elevated levels are encountered, the aircraft accident investigating authorities should take the following facts into consideration before arriving at any definite conclusions:

(a) How long did it take to retrieve the body?

(b) Was the blood exposed to the atmosphere and the sun? If so, for how long?

(c) How long was the blood stored in various conditions — ideal or otherwise?

Even if the body of victim is retrieved in a reasonable time and blood samples collected expeditiously, the samples should always be transferred to dark-coloured bottles, topped up with a layer of liquid paraffin, stored in refrigerated conditions and estimation carried out without delay.

Study of Soot Particles in Aircraft Fires

One of the main objectives of an air-crash investigation is to determine how long an individual survives a post-crash fire. Death can occur either during the flight, during the crash, or during the fire itself. Carboxyhaemoglobin provides insight into these possibilities. At the same time, it is important to know which materials burned and where. Thus, a parallel investigation concerns the soot particles that are found in the respiratory tract of the casualty.

Although in-flight fires are not very common, they cannot be ignored, given the threat of sabotage. Furthermore, an individual may survive the initial impact of the crash but may be too disabled to escape the vitiated atmosphere. The author has investigated an air crash in which an occupant died, with clear-cut evidence of ante-mortem burns when the aircraft crashed on the ground and caught fire. The autopsy showed that the deceased had fractures in both femur bones and no other significant injuries. The logical conclusion, therefore, was that he could not get out of the burning wreckage. Thus, survival in a toxic atmosphere gains importance and at the same time gives us an insight into the efficiency of rescue operations.

Chaturvedi[63] cited a study of 95 fire-related accidents that occurred worldwide over a 26-year period and involved about 2,400 fatalities. A significant number of fatalities had carboxyhaemoglobin levels of 20 per cent or more. This calls for the development of "combustion toxicology". In many developing countries, the presence of soot particles in the respiratory tract is merely noted and related to survival in a toxic atmosphere. Mitchelson[62] has detailed the use of electron spectroscopic imaging of such smoke particles to show that these particles have varied structure and composition. Birky[39] has suggested "computer interfaced pyrolysis mass spectrometry". Soot contains two portions. One is a high percentage of carbon while the other is a portion of the original polymer of the material which burnt to produce the soot. The above technique pyrolyses the soot into the ion source and the ion pattern thus obtained is analyzed on computer to identify the exact polymer which produced the soot. Thus, information is provided on the specific toxic material that burned and also on post-crash survival. The location of the deceased in the aircraft in relation to the source of fire can also assume importance when investigating the crash.

CHAPTER 3

ALCOHOL AND AVIATION

Before evaluating the effects of alcohol vis-à-vis aviation accidents, a pathologist must have basic knowledge on ethanol, its properties and effects on human physiology. The following paragraphs provide some basic information, as alcohol is often implicated in aircraft accidents. Note that the conventional word "alcohol" is used for ethanol.

Physical and Chemical Properties

As commonly used, the word "alcohol" refers to "ethanol" or grain alcohol/hydroxyl-ethane (C_2H_5OH). It has a boiling point of 78.3°C and a specific gravity of 0.79 at 20°C. It is a clear limpid fluid having a characteristic odour. It is completely miscible in water. The molecular weight of ethanol is 46, which is less than half that of the average amino acid and one-fourth that of glucose. Low molecular weight and high solubility allow it to diffuse rapidly through body membranes and into the tissues. It is more than twice as volatile as water. At concentrations below 20 per cent, alcohol in the body obeys Henry's law and, therefore, there is a constant ratio between the concentration of alcohol in the blood and in the alveolar air of lungs. The accepted alveolar–air: blood alcohol ratio is about 1: 2100.

Alcohol reduces oxidising agents and this property is utilised for its quantitative estimation. For example, potassium dichromate solution in the presence of sulphuric acid, when exposed to alcohol, will cause oxidation of alcohol to acetic acid with corresponding reduction of dichromate. Similarly, in the presence of DPN (di-phospho-pyridine nucleotide), the enzyme Alcohol Dehydrogenase (ADH) oxidises alcohol to acetaldehyde with the formation of an equivalent amount of reduced DPN (DPNH). It reacts with hot (105°C) Iodine Pentoxide, to form a proportional amount of Iodine vapours, which is also used as a technique in quantitative estimation.

Alcoholic Beverages

The consumption of alcohol is usually in the form of certain beverages containing mainly ethyl alcohol and water along with some flavouring agents. Vodka contains mainly water and alcohol and gin is flavoured with juniper berries or orange peels. Beer and ale contain dextrin along with alcohol. Wines contain sugar and certain essential oils are added to liquors.

Other substances automatically form in alcoholic beverages and are designated as congeners. Some of these are fusel oils (a mixture of propyl, butyl and other alcohols), organic acids, esters and acetaldehyde. Some wines and brandies contain traces of methyl alcohol due to the breakdown of the methyl group in grape pectin. Aged whiskey and brandy contain tannins and other compounds that are liberated from charred wood-barrels during "wooding" of the beverage.

Quantities of Alcohol in Beverages

Pathologists are often confronted with certain problems when alcohol is detected in the blood/tissue of aviation fatalities (aircrew). They have to work out the concentration of ethanol in the blood after the ingestion of alcoholic drinks, based upon circumstantial evidence. To do this, they must know the various concentrations of alcohol present in alcoholic drinks.

Usually, unless specified otherwise, beer contains 4 per cent to 6 per cent alcohol. Many ales have 5 per cent to 8 per cent and wines from 10 per cent to 20 per cent alcohol. Whiskey, brandy, gin, rum and vodka range from 40 per cent to 55 per cent alcohol. However, it is always necessary to find out which particular type of alcoholic drink the person had consumed and then work out the concentration in the blood.

The percentage of ethanol is usually not directly indicated on the labels of liquor bottles. For distilled beverages, alcohol is expressed as "proof". In the United States, 100 per cent proof means 50 per cent alcohol by volume.

In the United Kingdom, however, "proof" is used to denote 57 per cent alcohol by volume and in various brands alcohol concentration is designated by per cent proof or degree proof. For example, 25 UP (meaning 25 degrees under proof) means that the alcohol is 100 minus 25 (i.e. 75) degree proof. Thus, the alcohol concentration is 75 per cent of 57 per cent or 42.8 per cent alcohol by volume.

Most Indian brands of whiskey, rum and gin are 75 degree proof, or approximately 43 per cent alcohol by volume. Multiplication by 0.8 (the specific gravity of alcohol) will provide the amount in weight. For example, if concentration of alcohol in a beverage is 43 per cent, 100 ml of this beverage will contain 43 ml of alcohol. The weight of 43 ml alcohol would be 43 X 0.8 = 34.4 grams.

Alcohol on Ingestion

Absorption

Experimental data (obtained with ingestion of 24 per cent ethyl alcohol on an empty stomach) show that the absorption of alcohol is rapid in the stomach, duodenum and jejunum (about 50 per cent from the stomach itself). Alcohol absorption was 52 per cent in 15 minutes, 51–94 per cent in 30 minutes and practically complete within 2 hours. Absorption is supposed to be complete when the entire gastrointestinal tract reaches equilibrium with the remainder of the body. If the stomach is not fully empty, absorption is delayed, depending upon the quantum and type of food it contains.

Distribution

Alcohol is absorbed from the gastrointestinal tract and goes through portal circulation. Through general circulation, it finds its way to the right side of the heart and then to the lungs. As it establishes quick equilibrium with arterial blood, vascular organs such as the liver, kidneys and brain receive a higher quantity of alcohol at a quicker rate than do other organs. Soon after a few quick drinks, therefore, a person may feel tipsy and pass large quantities of urine. After storage equilibrium in various organs is achieved, the resultant concentration in all tissues is proportional to the water content of the tissue. Voluntary muscles have less blood flow per unit of weight as compared to vascular organs, like the brain. Thus, it takes about an hour for the former to attain equilibrium. As muscles form about 40 per cent of body weight, they finally take up an appreciable amount of alcohol with a corresponding decrease in brain, liver and kidney concentrations. This explains the sudden "sobering" which may occur after some time.

Most of the alcohol undergoes biochemical oxidation in the body to produce CO_2 and water. This is achieved by alcohol-dehydrogenase, which in the presence of co-enzyme diphosphopyridine nucleotide (DPN), produces acetaldehyde from alcohol, subsequently feeding Kreb's cycle with acetates. About 6 per cent of alcohol is excreted from the body unchanged through sweat, urine and breath. As the oxidation of alcohol proceeds at a constant rate, the rate of decrease in blood alcohol is also practically linear. Biochemical oxidation of alcohol starts in the liver, where alcohol, in the presence of DPN, catalyzed by ADH, is converted into acetaldehyde and reduced DPN (DPNH2). Soon after, acetaldehyde is converted to acetic acid by a complex enzyme mechanism in the liver itself. Acetic acid, in turn, reacts with body buffer salts to produce acetates. This happens so quickly that acetaldehyde usually disappears as fast as it is formed. Acetate is added to the body's acetate pool and is finally converted to CO_2 and water. Disulfuran (antabuse) and cyanamide retard the process of conversion of acetaldehyde to acetic acid and the resultant accumulation of acetaldehyde can produce an unpleasant "disulfuran effect".

Total body and blood alcohol level

As bones and fat have a lower concentration of water than blood, the blood level of alcohol is usually 17 per cent more than that of soft tissue. Widmark proposed the factor 'γ' to designate the ratio of alcohol concentration in body to alcohol concentration in the blood. This ratio averages 0.67 in men, with a range from 0.46 to 0.86. It is lower in women due to a larger amount of fatty tissue. This factor was obtained by giving a known amount of alcohol and obtaining the blood alcohol concentration curve over a period of several hours. As the curve is a straight line, one can extrapolate it back to the start, to calculate the level of blood alcohol which would have been achieved if no destruction or excretion had occurred. This gives the concentration of alcohol (denominator) in Widmark's formula. The numerator, of course, is obtained from the dose of alcohol and subject's body weight. The Widmark factor 'γ' can be used to approximately estimate, from the blood alcohol level and individual's body weight, the total quantity of alcohol in his body, at the time the blood sample was taken.

For example:
If the body weight of an individual is 150 lbs (70 kgs) and the blood alcohol concentration is 0.15 per cent (or 150 mg/100ml) then, as γ is 0.67 as defined in the previous paragraph:
Concentration in body/Concentration in blood = 0.67 or
Concentration in body/0.15 = 0.67
Thus, concentration in body = 0.67 x 0.15 = 0.1 per cent
0.1 per cent of 70 kg = 0.07 kg or 70 mg of alcohol.
70 mg will be contained in (70 x 10)/8 = 87 ml or 6 oz of 100 proof whiskey (57 per cent alcohol).

This represents unburnt alcohol remaining in the body. The person would have to drink more than 6 fluid ounces of 100 per cent proof whiskey to produce this level, as some alcohol will be eliminated during drinking, absorption and exercise etc. A simplified estimation of Widmark's 'γ' value by Forester's method is well documented and can be referred to if required.

The difference between whole blood and serum/plasma concentrations must be understood, as it is significant. Ethanol distributes within watery portions of body tissue and, therefore, it is logical that concentration will be more in plasma/serum than whole blood. Conversion of this is often done by using the logic that blood has a water content of about 86 per cent. Ethanol levels have thus been found to be higher in plasma/serum by 9–18 per cent. The recommended formula is as follows:

serum ethanol X 0.8 = whole blood ethanol
Whole blood ethanol / 0.8 = serum ethanol, or

Blood : Serum conversion is 1:1.2
Blood : Plasma conversion is 1: 1.2

Excretion of Alcohol in Urine

Administered orally, alcohol is quickly absorbed by simple diffusion from the gastro-intestinal tract. Peak concentration in the blood is achieved one half to two hours after ingestion. Alcohol level in the urine, however, reaches its peak 30 minutes later. Equilibrium between blood and urine is present when urine leaves the ureter. The water content of urine (approxtimately 97 ml/100 ml), exceeds that of blood by about 18 per cent. The commonly accepted figure for urine: blood alcohol is 1.25, meaning that urine contains a little less bound water than blood. An increase in the specific gravity of urine typically decreases this ratio.

It sometimes becomes necessary to work out the concentration of alcohol in the whole body given only the urine sample alcohol value. When doing so, certain facts must be remembered. The average concentration of alcohol in the blood is about 50 per cent higher than it is in the body as a whole. The level in urine is about 25 per cent above that in blood. Thus, 100 ml of urine will contain the alcohol in 100 X 1.5 X 1.25 = 187.5 or approx. 188 gm. of average body weight. This information is useful while calculating the amount of alcohol lost from the body after ingestion. Assuming that secretion of urine (stimulated by alcohol) is 3ml/minute or 180 ml/hour, the fraction of total body alcohol removed per hour from a 70 kg individual would be (1.88 X 180)/70 or 0.48 per cent. However, during the disappearance period, the body alcohol level is not constant but slowly drops to zero at a uniform rate. For this period, the average concentration of body alcohol is half of the initial level, so the average percentage removed per hour would be 0.24. Thus, with stated urine flow per kg of body-weight, and a single dose of administered alcohol, the percentage of dose lost in urine would be 0.24 times the disappearance period in an hour.

Related studies show the importance of estimating the ethanol in the urine of deceased aircrew members. Although the peak concentration of alcohol in the blood is achieved in 1/2 to 2 hours after ingestion, the alcohol level in urine reaches its peak about 30 minutes later as a part of the alcohol is excreted in urine unchanged. During the absorptive phase, blood alcohol levels are higher than those of urine. However, once absorption is complete and peak levels of ethanol develop in urine, the urinary concentration is always higher than that of blood and maintains a constant ratio till the end. Due to the concentration factor, alcohol levels of urine are always higher than those of blood and maintain a more or less constant ratio of 1.3:1. This observation has its own importance in aircraft accident investigation. Due to lingering traces of alcohol in urine, it may be possible to corroborate the evidence of a previous drinking bout, even when the ethanol level in the blood has declined to zero.

Evan and Jones showed in 1929 that the concentration of alcohol in urine provides an accurate indication of minimum quantity of alcohol consumed. Wyane[127] showed that once peak levels in urine are achieved, there is a good correlation between the levels of alcohol in samples of blood and those of urine taken half an hour later. The ratio usually accepted between urine and blood was 1.33:1. In his study, Froentjes[128] found this ratio to be 1.52:1. A special committee of the British Medical Association was set up for the purpose of working this out, and in the end suggested that the ratio is 1.32:1. Payne et al.[129] also confirmed this in 1966. With the advent of more accurate techniques, like gas-chromatography, Payne et al.[130] found the ratio to be 1.44:1. They were cautious lest this variation could lead to a miscarriage of justice, as most of these investigations were done in drunken driving cases.

Variability in this ratio (between 1.33:1 and 1.44:1) was partly attributed to the frequency of micturition in the post-absorptive phase, as reported by Walls.[131] Evidently, most of the work on this subject was undertaken with higher alcohol levels, the basic aim being prosecution of intoxicated drivers. Not many studies were done to establish this ratio in the lower range of alcohol levels. Studies in 1977 were undertaken using Indian subjects, as they may have different rate of ethanol metabolism due to racial variation (Bennion and Lynn[132]). During a study on "After-effects of alcohol on psycho-physiological functions in relation to flying performance of air crew" (AFMRC Project 423/71),[133] the author noticed that 9 hours after ingestion of alcohol, the blood ethanol levels declined to zero while some of the corresponding samples of urine continued to show traces.

This observation has important implications for aircraft accident investigations. If urine ethanol values continue to show higher figures than those of blood, a situation is likely to arise during the terminal phase of excretion, when blood will be free of alcohol with traces still present in the urine, indicating an ingestion of alcohol hours earlier. Adaval and Maruthi Ram[134] conducted a study on 86 healthy male volunteers. After ingestion of known quantities of alcohol and regulating the rate of drinking conventionally-used brands of rum and whiskey, blood and urine ethanol levels were estimated after 1/2, 1, 2, 4, 6, 9 and 12 hours. Mean urine: blood ethanol ratio was found to be 1.29: 1 (Standard deviation of plus-minus 0.23). After a period of 9 hours, no alcohol was detected in the blood whereas it was still present in several 9 and 12 hours samples of urine.

The importance of ethanol detection in urine is now being emphasised in relation to investigation of aircraft accidents as these observations can corroborate the evidence of a previous drinking bout. Urine, at the same time, is considered a better sample due to stable ethanol levels, and is less prone to contamination and decomposition.

Excretion of Alcohol in Breath, Urine and Faeces

Loss of alcohol in breath follows the same principle as in urine. It is 0.25 times the disappearance period in hours. As with urine, the loss would be less than the above figure where alcohol was administered in divided doses. Taking lung ventilation rate as 10 litres/minute in an individual weighing 70 kg, the loss would be

$$\frac{10 \times 60}{2 \times 70{,}000} \times 100 = 0.5\%$$

For the disappearance period, the average hourly loss would be half of this value, or 0.25 per cent.

The concentration of alcohol in sweat is the same as in urine. As the volume of sweat is about 50 per cent of urine output, it will be 0.2 per cent per hour for the disappearance period. In faeces, the loss of alcohol will depend on water content and is usually negligible.

Total Excretion

Total excretion thus will average 0.24 + 0.25 + 0.12 = 0.61 per cent per hour for the disappearance period. If this period is about 10 hours, approximately 6 per cent of the alcohol administered will be excreted. The disappearance period would result from the ingestion of about half a pint of average whiskey by an individual weighing 70 kg.

Measurement of Rate of Disappearance

The speed of decline of total body alcohol is usually inferred from the rate of decrease in blood alcohol level (after storage equilibrium is reached), assuming that '*r*' remains constant during the period. The curve for the phase of falling blood alcohol follows a straight-line course. Widmark proposed the factor 'beta' (β) to designate the drop in blood alcohol/minute expressed in parts per thousand. Thus, the calculated beta is in long decimal fractions. It is better to have it in milligrams per cent per hour (mg%/hour).

Another procedure is to measure the hourly drop in total body alcohol (mg/kg/hour). This is obtained by dividing the alcohol dosage in mg/kg by the disappearance time in hours. The average disappearance rate for a man is about 100 mg/kg/hour (range 55–186). The rate of disappearance (Widmark Factor β) is not altered by the concentration of alcohol, exercise or exposure to cold/heat or habituation. Because large variations in β occur regardless of drinking history, the differences observed in the limited number of subjects in experiments on habituation, might be due to inherent and not to acquired characteristics. Thus, β can be used to calculate blood alcohol concentration 2 hours earlier or so, assuming that there was no further drinking during the interval. Practically, the hourly drop in blood alcohol will range from 10–20 mg per cent with an average of 15 mg per cent (0.015 gm per cent). Thus, if blood alcohol was 0.174 per cent at a given time, the calculated figure 2 hours earlier would be between

0.194 per cent and 0.214 per cent (with an average of 0.204 per cent).

The average drop in total body alcohol is 100 mg/kg/hour. Hence a 70-kg person would dispose of 7 gm alcohol per hour, i.e. less than 2/3 ounce of 100 proof (50 per cent) whiskey. Six hours after drinking 1/2 pint (8 ounces, 240 ml or 4 pegs) of such whiskey, he would have oxidised or excreted the alcohol in is 6 X 2/3 = 4 oz. (120 ml) of whiskey and he would be alcohol-free in 12 hours (12×2 divided by 3 = 8 oz. in about 12 hours). Here are some examples:

Q. A 70-kg person has taken 3 large pegs of whiskey. When he will be alcohol free?

A. Rate of disappearance in a 70-kg individual is 7 gm/hour (or 2/3 oz. of 100 proof whiskey).

3 large pegs will be 180 ml or 6 oz. of alcohol

So, 2/3 oz. in 1 hour and 1 oz. in 3/2 hour

And thus, 6 oz. in 3/2×6 = 9 hours.

The average drop of total body alcohol is 100 mg/kg/hour or 0.1 gm/kg/hour. In a 70-kg individual it is 7 gm/hour (or 2/3 oz. of 100-proof whiskey). As 2/3 oz. is 20 ml, it will be 20 ml of liquor (approx. 43 per cent alcohol)/hour. A 70-kg individual will lose 120 ml or two large pegs in 6 hours, and will lose 240 ml (4 large pegs) in 12 hours.

Effects of Ethanol

Ethyl-alcohol is the main constituent of alcohol beverages that affect human systems, and so the following discussion will focus on these effects.

The Skin

Ingestion of a moderate amount of alcohol causes vasodilatation. This effect is central in origin and is responsible for "flushed face" and general hyperaemia. As skin contains temperature-sensitive nerve endings, hyperaemia creates a feeling of warmth although there is no rise in body temperature. There is some increase in perspiration. In profound alcohol intoxication, however, the skin is pale and clammy due to impaired circulation.

The Gastrointestinal tract

Alcohol causes a temporary increase of gastric acidity. Only mucosa of the stomach-antrum and duodenum are alcohol sensitive in stimulating acid secretion by gastric glands throughout the stomach. As intravenous administration of ethanol also causes increased gastric acidity, it is logical to consider this as a central phenomenon. Alcohol concentration above 15 per cent causes irritation and inflammation of gastric mucosa. Vomiting usually occurs after heavy drinking when blood alcohol levels are usually above 120 mg/100 ml. This action is also central in origin, as demonstrated by the administration of intravenous ethanol. In the small intestines, alcohol is absorbed quickly and its concentration is not high enough to cause any effects other than a mild transient increase in secretions.

The Circulatory system

Oral ingestion of 40 ml of whiskey increases heart rate, blood pressure and total blood flow. These effects usually last for 30 minutes. No definite effect on coronary circulation has been established. In severe alcoholic intoxication, a marked fall in blood pressure with a quick and low volume pulse has been observed.

The Liver

Alcohol damage to the liver has been well documented. Loss of glycogen and increased urinary copro-porphyrins-3 have been demonstrated. Incidence of cirrhosis is 6 times more in alcoholics, due to direct toxic effects as well as the nutritional deficiency so commonly encountered in chronic alcoholics. Fatty changes in the liver are often encountered during routine histopathological studies conducted on aircrew aviation fatalities. Though not directly responsible for accident, these findings give us an insight into the pilot's general health as well as his vulnerability to fat embolism.

The Kidneys

Alcohol causes high urinary output. This is partly due to increased water intake but is mostly due to the diuretic effect of alcohol. As the kidney is a highly vascular organ, initially its share of alcohol in the blood is high. At the same time, alcohol causes inhibition in the production of anti-diuretic hormone by the pituitary.

The Central Nervous System

Alcohol is a depressant and not a "stimulant", as generally believed. An apparent stimulant-like action is a result of depression of restraining mechanisms. Alcohol causes deterioration in the finer grades of attention, judgment, reflection and ability to comprehend. This explains the typical behaviour of a person under the influence of alcohol. Soldiers become more "courageous" as they do not comprehend danger and do not reflect on it. A speaker is not tormented and influenced by the surrounding public and thus speaks freely and animatedly. One's self-appraisal rises greatly.

The depressant effect of alcohol can be considered in three areas:

1. Lessened efficiency of vision and hearing: Studies conducted by using a "flicker fusion apparatus" show that visual impairment occurs at different blood alcohol levels. Minimum levels to show this deterioration in occasional, moderate and heavy drinkers are 10–20 mg/100 ml, 20–30 mg/100 ml and 40–70 mg/100 ml respectively (Kumar et al.[133]). Alcohol has the same effect on vision as setting a gray glass in front of the eyes or driving with sunglasses in twilight. With respect to hearing, it has been established that after alcohol ingestion, higher tone intensity is required to perceive a given tone or to differentiate between tones.
2. Impaired coordination of voluntary muscles: Even before obvious signs of drunkenness, like a staggering gait and slurred speech, efficiency of coordination in performing intricate muscular movements is significantly reduced. This is true even after ingestion of a small amount of alcohol. There is a significant deterioration in the performance of tasks such as typewriting, handwriting, drawing, target practice, arm-steadiness and driving, even with blood alcohol levels as low as 10–20mg/100ml. Reaction time is increased by 10–30 per cent, which can be hazardous, especially during an emergency.

3. Deterioration of judgment and self-control: Alcohol-induced euphoria and loss of inhibition are well known. Inflated ego and over-confidence lead people to take chances that they would normally prefer to avoid. Such subjective behaviour cannot be measured and quantified as individuals vary in their response and have varying degrees of "tolerance". However, a study conducted on a large number of subjects has shown that with blood alcohol levels below 50 mg/100 ml, very few persons were "drunk". However, many more showed "drunkenness" with levels between 50 and 100 mg/100 ml and almost all were "drunk" with levels above 200 mg/100 ml. Higher tolerance in some individuals can be either inherent or acquired. However, one can generally anticipate the influence of alcohol vis-à-vis alcohol levels in blood as highlighted by certain authors,[135] and shown in Table 3.1.

Table 3.1

Whiskey (oz.)	**Blood Concentration** (mg/100 ml)	**Influence**
1–2	10–15	None to mild euphoria
3–4	50–100	Mild influence on stereoscopic vision & dark adaptation
4–6	100–150	Euphoria, loss of inhibition, prolonged reaction time
6–7	150–200	Moderately severe poisoning, reaction-time greatly prolonged, loss of inhibition, slight disturbance in equilibrium & coordination
8–9	200–250	Severe degree of poisoning, disturbance of equilibrium & coordination, retarded thought process, clouding of consideration
10–15	250–400	Deep, possibly fatal, coma

Alcohol Estimation in Biological Samples

Collection and Preservation of Samples

The samples usually analyzed for alcohol include blood, urine, saliva and breath in living subjects. While conducting autopsies, samples like blood, urine, organs, muscles and stomach contents are usually preserved for estimation of alcohol. Body organs can be stored in the refrigerator. It should be ensured that formaldehyde does not contaminate the samples. It is worth remembering that many embalming fluids contain formaldehyde and methanol. Putrefied tissues are generally unsuitable as they lose alcohol (if present) with time and at the same time produce spurious alcohol as a by-product of putrefaction (Canfield, Kupiec and Huffine;[136] and Kalant[137]). Separation of alcohol from body tissues is achieved either by distillation or desiccation in a Widmark blood alcohol flask. When the sample is found to contain ethanol, it may be difficult to know whether it is due to post-mortem formation or to genuine ingestion. Recently, Johnson et al.[138] utilised the urinary 5 HTOL/5 HIAA (5-hydroxytryptophol/5-hydroxy indole acetic acid) ratio to differentiate between genuine alcohol ingestion and post-mortem formation of ethanol when results of biological samples are positive.

When taking a blood sample from a vein of a living subject, ensure that the skin is not cleaned with an alcohol-containing substance. Blood should be collected in a screw-capped bottle with sodium fluoride as an anticoagulant. There should be as little air space in the bottle as possible. Refrigeration/preservation in ice is recommended. (Urine and saliva samples can also be preserved in screw-capped bottles and refrigerated.)

While taking a breath sample, ensure that there is no trace of alcoholic drink in the subject's mouth, as this will give an erroneous result. The mouth should be thoroughly rinsed with water before collecting the breath sample. Breath is usually analyzed immediately but can be stored for an hour or two in a polyvinyl chloride bag or an aluminum pouch.

Estimation

Many estimation procedures are non-specific, as they cannot differentiate between various types of alcohol.[139-142] Methods that are specific to ethanol are recommended for fatal aircraft accident investigation.

Chemical methods commonly employed are "dichromate methods". Many of these are semi-quantitative, based upon the fact that potassium dichromate solution in concentrated sulphuric acid changes colour from yellow to greenish blue when an alcoholic solution is bubbled through it at room temperature. Alcohol is oxidised to acetic acid and valence of chromium changes.

Widmark methods are also based on the property of ethanol to reduce dichromate with the resultant colour change measured colorimetrically. This reaction is relatively non-specific and occurs with a number of other reducing agents that might be present in physiological fluids. (These agents include acetone, ketone and aldehyde; as well as intermediate products of metabolism of some drugs, like salicylic acid.) Alcohol, other than ethanol, will also give a positive reaction. Accordingly, preliminary tests should be carried out to exclude these substances. These methods are relatively time-consuming and uneconomical in terms of laboratory staff. On the other hand, they are reliable and accurate in competent hands. The Widmark method or a modification thereof is still a commonly used procedure in forensic laboratories of developing countries. Both micro and macro methods are available (Gradwohl's Legal Medicine[143]). The Kozelka and Hine dichromate method has also been recommended (Todd & Sanford[139]) with alkaline mercuric oxide treatment of the first distillate. This method has a recovery of 96–98 per cent of the alcohol from blood samples and a standard error of +/-8 mg per cent.

Gas

Chromatographic methods are very specific and accurate as they can separate fractions of various types of alcohol. The author[134] has used a dual-column gas-chromatograph fitted with flame ionisation detector. Copper columns of 4 metres in length and 0.6 cm in diameter were filled with 10 per cent polyethylene glycol-400 coated on celite 100–120 mesh. Temperatures of the injector, columns and detector were regulated at 130, 90 and 110 degrees Centigrade, respectively. Nitrogen was used as the carrier gas at a flow rate of 45 ml/minute. This technique was modified from the one advocated by Curry et al.[141] The HPLC Method has also been tried. Although high-pressure liquid chromatography can be used to detect and quantify ethanol, this technique is normally available only in sophisticated laboratories.

Estimation of Ethanol in Breath Samples

The procedure for collecting breath samples has already been described. Estimation is based on the assumption that the distribution of alcohol between blood and alveolar air obeys Henry's law. That is, the blood-to-alveolar-air alcohol ratio is close to 2100:1 for the temperature at which breath leaves the nose/mouth. Thus, when the blood contains 100mg/100 ml alcohol, the exhaled air will contain 100 mg of alcohol in 210 litres of breath.

Several instruments are available for the detection and quantification of ethanol in breath. At one time, Harger's Drunkometer, based upon the oxidation of acidified potassium permanganate, was used. Breath passed through the reagent made the purple colour disappear if it contained alcohol. Similarly, Forrester's Intoxicometer and Greenberg and Keator's Alcometer were once used. With the advent of more sophisticated instruments, however, both methods have been discarded.

Since the mid 1980s, infrared® technology has been utilised, which is more specific due to the use of many optical filters. A narrow selected band of infrared light is passed through one side of a breath sample chamber. As the light emerges from the other side, absorbance of infrared is noted and alcohol concentration is measured by Lambert-Beer law. The result is calculated in comparison to that obtained against a known concentration of ethanol vapour.

Fuel Cell Technology is another method to detect alcohol in the breath. An alcohol fuel cell consists of a porous, chemically inert layer coated on both sides with finely divided platinum (platinum-black). The porous layer is impregnated with an acidic electrolyte solution and applies platinum wire electric connections to platinum black surfaces. A gas inlet is provided for entry of breath. As alcohol-containing breath enters, there is an alcohol-oxidation reaction. A fixed number of electrons are freed per molecule of alcohol. Oxidation occurs in the upper surface of the fuel cell and freed $H+$ ions migrate to the lower surface and combine with atmospheric oxygen to form water, consuming one electron per $H+$ ion. Thus, the upper surface has excess electrons and the lower surface has a corresponding lesser number. If the two surfaces are connected electrically, current will flow to obtain equilibrium and this current will indicate the amount of alcohol consumed by the fuel cell. Proper calibration will indicate directly the breath alcohol concentration.

Blood Alcohol and Aircrew Performance

Performance decrements resulting from alcohol are extensively recorded in the literature.[144-148] As noted earlier, self-control, judgment, muscular coordination and discretion often deteriorate even with the consumption of a small amount of alcohol. Visual and auditory sensations are also known to suffer.

The effects of ethanol assume greater significance when the subject is engaged in a complex task such as flying. With the advent of complicated high performance aircraft, a pilot's physical and mental efficiency is required to be at a peak. Factors like acceleration forces and vestibular sensations demand a great deal from the aircrew. Psychomotor performances under such situations also have to be extremely efficient.

The literature is replete with research on the effects of alcohol on skilled performance. Earlier studies were related to alcohol vis-à-vis driving ability. As early as 1954, however, Askness[149] demonstrated that levels of alcohol far below the commonly accepted legal limits had adverse effects upon flying skills. Harper and William[152] supported this view. In 1973, Billing's report[150] was published, which recorded tracking data and procedural errors in instrument-rated pilots under the influence of 0.04, 0.08 and 0.12 per cent blood alcohol concentrations, and found marked decrement in performance at all levels, thus narrowing down the lower limit to 40 mg per cent. In 1977, Henry[151] studied psychomotor performance in an automated system around a link Flight Trainer and showed that even 25 mg per cent blood alcohol levels caused significant performance decrement. Kumar[133] studied Indian Air Force subjects by conducting Flight Oriented Psychomotor Tests, Critical Fusion Frequency, Stability of Attention and Choice Reaction Time tests and demonstrated that even 12 hours after ingestion of 180 ml of conventional whiskey/rum, there was significant performance deterioration though blood ethanol levels had declined to zero.

Alcohol has been incriminated in a large number of fatal aircraft accidents. In the past four decades, many reports have been published, some of the earliest being those of Harper and William,[152] Mohler,[153–154] Ryan and Mohler,[155] Alha and Tamminen,[156] Davis,[157, 158] and Zeller[159]. Most of these earlier reports indicated a constant rate of occurrence but detailed analyses showed that in most cases, the relationship was associated or contributory and not causal (Cullen, Drysdale and Mayes[23]). Toxicological findings in Federal Aviation Administration general accidents wherein 377 FAA aviation fatalities were investigated showed ethanol levels of more than 10 mg per cent were found in 14.8 per cent of cases but only 4.5 per cent were determined to be due to ethanol ingestion (Kuhlman, Levine, Smith and Hordinsky[120]).

As acute effects of alcohol on skilled performance are very well known, many countries enforce the rule specifying a "bottle to throttle" interval. In the US Air Force, this interval is 8 hours between alcohol consumption and flying, whereas in India, the Air Staff Instructions require a period of 12 hours. The quantity of alcohol permitted is, however, not specified. A question often asked is what level of alcohol is "safe" as far as flying is concerned. A simple and categorical answer is "no level of alcohol is safe"! As seen in the studies conducted by Kumar et al.,[133] performance decrement was observed even after blood ethanol levels had declined to zero. Cook[160] has provided a review of research regarding aircrew alcohol consumption, impairment of performance due to alcohol and incidence of aviation accidents attributable to alcohol consumption by aircrews. He has highlighted that performance decrement may be present even though blood alcohol levels decline to zero and so many accidents, though actually due to alcohol consumption, may be erroneously reported as negative.

CHAPTER 4

PROBLEMS OF DRUG DETECTION BY ROUTINE AND SPECIALISED TECHNIQUES

Detecting a drug in biological samples is one of the most difficult and challenging objectives of analytical science. As the requirements have become more and more precise and difficult, the challenge is being met by improving the technology. At this juncture, we have come to a stage where drug assay has become the domain of an exclusive group of analytical biochemists who have devoted their lives to this topic.

To a layman, the detection of drugs in the blood or urine might appear to be accomplished easily by conducting some chemical tests in a standard clinical laboratory. This belief is based upon the fact that in earlier days, chemical analyzers were used to detect drugs and poisons that were administered in lethal doses for suicidal and homicidal purposes. The huge amounts of drugs or poison present in such cases made detection and analysis easy to perform.

When a drug is administered in a therapeutically controlled dosage, however, the concentrations in biological (blood and urine) samples are very minute. These traces cannot be detected or quantified by conventional means applicable to clinical chemistry (Blackmore[161]). Some drugs may have chemical configurations similar to the natural ingredients of blood, making them almost impossible to distinguish. Many interfering substances also make detection difficult. Concentrations in blood and urine keep fluctuating according to dosage schedule and the sensitivity of the test may not be adequate to detect the lowest concentrations. Finally, many drugs metabolise quickly and are excreted in urine in the form of simple organic substances that are normally present. For these reasons, the examination of urine for detection of these drugs may prove futile.

One can still apply these simple chemical tests if one knows the nature of drug that was likely to have been administered. However, it is not possible to process a sample for all possible drugs that might have been taken. Many accidents that are caused by human failure may be due to drugs taken clandestinely without informing the authorized medical attendant. Thus, therapeutic levels of these drugs and their metabolites are required to be detected in biological samples. Emphasis is laid on detection of metabolites of these drugs by sensitive techniques but non-availability of metabolite reference standards, endogenous substance interference and low tissue levels render the analysis difficult (Chaturvedi and Canfield[162]).

Selective serotonin reuptake inhibitors (SSRIs) are often prescribed for depression. These drugs are notorious for causing performance decrement. Furthermore, they tend to interact with other drugs, alcohol and hypoxia, to cause adverse effects. Akin and Chaturvedi[163] report that out of 4,184 fatal civil accidents investigated at the Civil Aerospace Medical Institute there were 61 accidents in which SSRIs were detected in members of the aircrew. Commonly used medicines were fluoxetine, sertraline, peroxetine and citalopram. Other drugs, like analgesics, sympathomimetics and ethanol were also detected, which could have had contributory effects in at least 9 cases.

Chaturvedi and Canfield[162] point out that when the drugs contained in the samples result from therapeutic and sub-therapeutic doses, it is necessary to determine the presence of the parent drug as well as its metabolites. These metabolites may be chemically reactive, physiologically active or inactive, the latter two of which cannot be determined. Even though very sophisticated techniques are available, there are still limitations, such as a paucity of metabolite reference standards, endogenous interference and low tissue metabolite levels. It is encouraging that in spite of these drawbacks, some drugs and their metabolites can be detected, including terfenadine, cocaine, diazepam, temazepam and oxazepam. In testing regimens, AFIP[34] distinguishes between drugs of abuse (amphetamines, barbiturates, benzodiazepines, cannabinoids, cocaine, opiates and phencyclidine) and others (acetaminophen, antidepressants, antihistamines, chloroquine, dextromethorphan, lidocaine, mefloquine, narcotic analgesics, phenothiazines, phenytoin, salicylates, verapamil etc).

A brief review of commonly used procedures will help to understand the evolution of this discipline.[164,165]

Screening Chemical Tests

These tests are based upon the action of some chemical compounds on drugs to produce either a coloured precipitate or a coloured solution. Such methods, developed during the early days of toxicology, were mainly used in cases of suspected suicide or homicide. They were carried out directly on blood or urine samples or gastric aspirates and were restricted to only some of the known agents (alcohol, salicylates, chlorpromazine, phenothiazides, aminophenols and carboxyhaemoglobin). Furthermore, they were used only when there was strong suspicion of a particular drug or poison. However, the tests were not at all sensitive to detect the drugs in the small concentrations achieved with therapeutic doses.

Extraction Procedures

To overcome this difficulty, extraction procedures were employed in which specimens of blood, urine or stomach contents were processed to obtain extracts. These extracts were acid-ether and alkaline chloroform, depending upon the suspected drug. Extracts were dried and the residue was subjected to either simple chemical colorimetric tests or was evaluated by measuring the maximum absorption of light at different wavelengths, including ultraviolet range. Common drugs estimated by these techniques include *acid extracts* (Barbiturates, Diazepam, Ergot alkaloids, Glutethemides, Methaquilone and Salicylic acid) and *alkaline extracts* (Amitriptyline, Amphetamines, Codeine, Meprobromate, Phenytoin and Quinine).

Extraction methods are still employed in a number of toxicological laboratories. To be useful, however, they must be capable of dealing with a wide variety of samples, efficient enough to detect low concentrations, and applicable to a large number of different substances. Although substitutions of colorimeters with spectrophotometers increased the sensitivity of tests, the elaborate extraction procedures were open to question and vulnerable to a large number of variables. No single method was found to be suitable for all samples. The main object here was detection and not quantitative analysis. Consequently, the minimal concentrations obtained due to therapeutic administration of drugs went undetected.

Chromatography

Chromatographic procedures are based on one or more of the four physicochemical principles: adsorption, partition, ion exchange and exclusion. Techniques such as column chromatography, paper chromatography, thin layer chromatography and gas chromatography developed from these principles.

Chromatography is used to separate or purify small amounts of closely related compounds from one another in a mixture. The system has two phases. In the *stationary* phase, a liquid or solid is fixed or motionless during the process. In the *mobile* phase, a liquid or gas moves through the system. Four possible systems involving mobile and stationary phases are liquid-liquid, gas-liquid, liquid-solid and gas-solid. Chromatography represents a dynamic system of mobile and stationary phases that blend as an inter-phasing operation, which is changing continuously.

When the physicochemical process of partitioning is involved, it is referred to as "partition chromatography". This consists of liquid–liquid or gas–liquid phases. This principle is used in column chromatography, paper chromatography and thin layer chromatography. The principle of adsorption is used in column chromatography, gas chromatography and thin-layer chromatography.

Column Chromatography

This procedure uses tubular columns that are packed with sorbents such as charcoal or inert particles coated with a stationary liquid. The sample is introduced into the column and an appropriate solvent system is allowed to wash through the column. The material that emerges will be a solvent containing separated compounds in the elutes, which are serially collected. Under identical conditions, the same compounds will always take the same amount of time to elute from a particular column. This "elution time" or "retention time" can be used as method of identification, either by referring to the time or by comparing it with a known substance. Thus, separation and identification are both achieved.

Paper Chromatography

This procedure involves a combination of adsorption and partition as the medium is a cellulose matrix containing entrapped water. The sample is applied as a liquid spot, a few centimetres from one edge of a filter paper and allowed to dry. The solvent is then allowed to flow over it. The mobile liquid phase of the solvent here moves by capillary action over the sample, causing separation of its components into individual spots on the filter paper. The unit of measurement is Rf, a fraction that equals the distance that a sample component travels (in cm) divided by the distance (in cm) the solvent front has traveled. Under identical conditions, the Rf of a particular compound is constant. Therefore, if the Rf is known, the substance can be identified by referring to a table in which the values of all compounds are provided. In case of doubt, a known substance is run as a control which should give the same Rf value. To visualise separated compounds, the paper must be sprayed with the appropriate stain and the compounds then quantified densitometrically or by elution. Visualisation of separated fractions can be done by exposure to ultraviolet light, where many compounds can be revealed as fluorescent or absorbing spots.

Many modifications and sophistications have been achieved and various systems have been recommended for groups of drugs including barbiturates, carbamates, dicoumerols, organo-phosphorous compounds, salicylates, steroids and thiazides. However, the procedures are not as simple as they might appear. Two-dimensional paper chromatography equipment, meticulous control of internal and external environment and perfect equilibration with vapour are prerequisites for achieving accurate results. Simply calculating the Rf value and referring to tables to identify the drugs is not recommended unless the Rf value of each component is established in one's own laboratory. Even then, it may be necessary to run a large number of controls parallel to the test samples. Experience in this field is necessary to achieve desired results. Even then, the time element to isolate and identify drugs is considerable.

Thin-Layer Chromatography

To achieve speed of detection, higher sensitivity and greater resolution, the use of paper chromatography has shifted to thin layer chromatography (TLC). This is similar to paper chromatography but usually employs the chromatographic principles of adsorption (liquid–solid) for separating most non-polar material. It is more versatile, faster and sensitive. It permits a choice of adsorbents like alumina gel (which has higher adsorption than silica gel activated), diatomaceous earth (celite or Kieselguhr) or cellulose powder. Silica gel is acidic as well as active and is universal in use. Alumina is basic and useful to separate bases and steroids. Celite is neutral and inactive, often being used to separate sugars and pharmaceuticals.

Glass plates are thinly and uniformly coated with a slurry of one of these materials, dried, and then activated by heating and stored in a desiccator. The mixture of components to be separated is applied quantitatively in a suitable solvent, as small spots. The bottom of the plate is placed in the solvent system, which moves gradually up the thin layer. The plate is then removed, air dried and examined for separated components. Visualisation of resolved components is achieved by: (a) spraying the plate with corrosives such as acids, (b) spraying with colour developing system (c) exposure to short wave UV (254 nm) to detect chromato-spots as non-fluorescing black spots or (d) exposure to long wave (350–366 nm) UV light to excite fluorescence.

The basic measurement is the same as it is for paper chromatography (Rf values). Identification by comparison with known standards is preferable to simply noting the Rf values. By using suitable standards, semi-quantitative methods can be developed.

Besides higher speed, sensitivity and resolution, TLC can use material as little as 0.1 microgram (μg) for analysis as compared with at least 10 to 20 μg by other methods. However, elution and quantification of separated components from a thin layer plate is a difficult and cumbersome procedure. Equipment became increasingly sophisticated over time, and many systems now provide the material as well as Rf values. These can separate and detect substances such as nitrogenous bases, anti-histaminics, phenothiazines, narcotic analgesics, ergot alkaloids, barbiturates and allied compounds, cardiac glycosides, aspirin, salicylates, corticosteroids, estrogens, vitamins and sulphonamides.

Although the actual procedure of separation takes only one to two hours, detection and quantification are cumbersome. "Instant Thin-Layer Chromatography" has now been developed and is faster, though less sensitive.

Gas Chromatography

This procedure is similar to partition chromatography but utilises an inert gas in place of the mobile liquid phase. It is based on adsorption and partition chromatographic principles. In gas–solid chromatography, there is an inert carrier gas as the mobile phase and the sorbent is a solid of large surface (e.g. charcoal). In gas–liquid chromatography, the mobile phase is the same gas but the sorbent is a non-volatile liquid coated on an inert solid support such as silica gel on celite particles. The stationary phase is packed in steel columns and the mobile phase passes through these to develop equilibrium. The columns are heated to a desired temperature. Then, when the sample is injected into the column, ingredients of the sample volatalise and pass out from the other end of the column at different times. Each component has its own retention time under standard conditions. By using a detector, components coming out from the column one by one each record a peak on the recording paper. Each component can be quantified by comparing the peaks with those obtained after injecting a known quantity of the same compound (Curry et al.[141]).

Virtually any substance that boils without decomposition, or that can yield a volatile stable derivative, can be subjected to gas chromatographic analysis. Steroids, alcohol, barbiturates and anticonvulsants can be easily separated and quantified. Various assemblies have been recommended that have flame-ionisation and thermal conductivity detectors. However, assemblies with electron capture detectors are used in most laboratories. Uniform column packing, correct temperature control of columns and the computerisation of peaks on the recorder are necessary. This technology takes some infrastructure and much experience to establish itself. Even then, non-volatile substances and metallic elements cannot be detected by this technique.

High Performance Liquid Chromatography

Since the early 1970s the development of pumps, columns, flow monitors and other instrumentation has allowed aqueous or organic solutions to be pumped through columns with pressure between 500 and 5,000 pounds per square inch. In addition, controlled pore size porous glasses for size-exclusion chromatography have been developed and totally spherical glass beads with very small sizes of 60, 100, 500 and 1,000 angstroms are commercially available. Very carefully controlled spherical silica gel beads of the same size are also available for adsorption chromatography. As different molecules absorb differently, separation can be achieved in a few minutes using the same type of solvents as used for silica gel TLC. The disadvantage of adsorption chromatography with HPLC is that the extent of hydration of silica gel, which is critically important, continues to change as various amounts of solvents are pumped through the columns. Consequently, exact reproduction of separating conditions is difficult and equilibration time may be prolonged.

One further development is "reverse phase" column packing, which involves covalent bonding of octadecyl silane (ODS) to small porous spherical glass beads. An-ion and cat-ion exchange-coated glass beads are also available commercially.

Detection is based upon the same principle as Gas Liquid Chromatography. The suspected drug is run through the appropriate column and separated out. Identification is based upon its retention time, which is further confirmed by running a fixed quantity of a known drug as a control. The quantification of peaks on the recorder is automatically achieved by computerisation.

The entire HPLC system is a full-fledged laboratory in which completely automated and computerised procedures are involved. The reagents have to be of specific spectroscopic grades and should be purified by milli-pore filters. A large number of prepared columns are available for specific groups of drugs. A high degree of expertise must be developed in this field by continuous exposure of workers to this discipline. Other variants of chromatography, such as Instant Thin Layer Chromatography, Ion-exchange Chromatography, Gel-permeation (size-exclusion) Chromatography and Affinity Chromatography, are not discussed in this chapter.

Immunoassay

When many living organisms are exposed to a foreign substance, called an antigen, they produce antibodies that react specifically with that antigen. This response takes place if the antigen is either a macromolecule such as a protein or polysaccharide of molecular weight greater than 1,000, or a more complex organism such as a red blood cell. Thus, in order to produce antibodies specific to smaller moieties like certain drugs, it is necessary to couple them chemically to a carrier. Typical carriers include Bovine Serum Albumin (BSA), Key Hole Limpet Hemocyanin (KHL) and synthetic polypeptides.

Haptene combines with a carrier to form Haptene Carrier Conjugate. When injected into suitable animals, it produces anti-haptene-carrier antibodies, which are extracted to produce anti-haptene anti-serum.

Haptene must be joined to the conjugate in such a way that the conformation of haptene stays unchanged and its active functional groups remain accessible. The choice of animal has to be restricted to a species that is a genetic responder to the carrier and haptene. There should be minimal variations in response between individuals within a species (a problem that has not been fully overcome). Crude sera is purified by standard immunological methods. Alternatively, selective precipitation with electrolytes/ethanol, column chromatography based on molecular sieves or ion-exchange chromatography can be used.

Once produced and purified, anti-sera can be used as reagent in a number of detection processes right from simple and elegant hemagglutination-inhibition assay to the sophisticated electron-spin immunoassay.

If a fixed amount of antibody is mixed with a known amount of antigen, which is labelled in a suitable way, an equilibrium is set up. The addition of unlabelled antigen will result in displacement of bound antigen.

A drug is labelled with an enzyme, then mixed with a drug antibody. As a result of this conjugation, activity of the enzyme is reduced. When a sample containing a drug is introduced in this combination, this drug (which is unlabelled) will compete and release the labelled drug from the combination. This will trigger activity in the enzyme and this activity will be proportional to the amount of drug present in the sample.

For this procedure, serum has to be stored at 2 to 8 degrees Centigrade. It is necessary that it should not be hemolysed or lipemic. Levels depend upon the last dose of drug taken and mode of administration, etc. Multiple specimens may be needed to confirm the results.

Radioimmunoassay

In this method, the proportion of bound and unbound drug is detected by using radio-tagging. Labelling of antigen is achieved by replacing an atom in the molecule by a radioactive one. Three isotopes are commonly used: C14, I125 and Tritium 3H. Tritium 3H and C14 emit beta radiation while I125 emits gamma- and X-rays. The choice is dictated by the particular circumstances that prevail in the laboratory concerned. In order to measure relative amounts of free and bound radio-labelled antigen, the two components should be separated. The separation process has to be rapid and complete so that mass-action equilibrium between antigen and antibody is not disturbed. Several methods can be used:

(a) Precipitation of antibody-bound drug with an electrolyte or organic solvent followed by filtration or ultracentrifugation.
(b) Adsorption of free drug by charcoal followed by filtration and ultracentrifugation.
(c) A double antibody technique. This procedure uses a second antibody raised against globulins of the animals in which the first antibody was produced. The second antibody precipitates the drug antibody

complex, followed by the usual filtration and centrifugation.

(d) Solid phase adsorption. An antibody specific to the drug under analysis is either adsorbed or chemically bound to the inside walls of plastic tubes used as analytical vessels. Alternatively, it can be attached to Sephadex, which is added to the reaction medium. After equilibrium, the unbound drug remains in solution and can be separated.

(e) Filtration through a nitro-cellular membrane, which retains the antigen-antibody complex and yields a filtrate containing only the free drug.

Radioactivity of each sample is measured in terms of counts per minute, corrected for background count rate. One sample without separation of free and bound drug is used to give a reference value of 100 per cent, and the remaining samples and results are expressed in terms of a percentage of this value against concentration or logarithm of this quantity.

Enzyme Inhibition Immunoassay

For an enzyme to act on its substrate, the substrate should have free access to the site of action of the enzyme. If this access is impeded, the enzymatic reaction does not take place or occurs very slowly. As an example, consider the enzyme "lysozyme". Tag a morphine molecule near its active site. Now, anti-morphine antibodies are brought in contact with this complex. There will be no enzyme activity, as the access to the site of lysozyme activity is blocked. Now if we add free morphine, this morphine will displace the bound morphine and free the enzyme to act. The activity of the enzyme will be directly proportional to the amount of drug (in this case, morphine) present in the tested sample. This method avoids the separation of stages inherent in the radio-immunoassay. Various systems have been developed to monitor and quantify enzymatic activity. Due to difficulties encountered in obtaining a highly reproducible light scattering system, G6PDH is being used to measure changes in optical density at 340 nm. These kits are available commercially.

Haemagglutination Inhibition

Tanned red cells of sheep are coated with the conjugate of rabbit serum and drug. Antiserum raised against the drug is incubated with an unknown material at room temperature for 10 minutes, and a suspension of coated RBC is added. After further incubation of 90–120 minutes, cells are examined for haemagglutination. If the drug is present in sufficient concentration in the unknown (tested) material, drug antibodies in the antiserum react with this and none is left over to agglutinate the indicator RBCs. This method can be made semi-quantitative by taking serial dilutions of the antiserum.

Latex Agglutination Inhibition Immunoassay

Molecules of the drug under test can be adsorbed on the latex particles. When suspended, they produce a milky white homogeneous appearance. When in contact with the appropriate antiserum, the latex particles are agglutinated and leave a clear supernatant. The serum or urine sample is incubated with the antiserum. Then the antigen-latex complex is added. If the sample contains an antigen, it will combine with the antibodies and so the latter will not remain free. As a result, the latex particles will remain unagglutinated. This method is easy to perform and gives clear-cut negative and positive results. However, it is non-quantitative.

Other Methods

Certain techniques like Flame Photometry, Mass Spectrometry and Atomic Absorption Spectro-photometry are not discussed here as they are used only to detect metallic substances.

Summary

It is difficult to enumerate the merits and demerits of various analytical procedures. When we evaluate these methods in relation to our requirements, however, it is evident that the usual chemical screening and extraction methods are not adequate to detect trace quantities of various drugs in human biological samples. This is particularly true when the exact nature of the drug taken is not known a priori. Even if there is a strong suspicion of a particular drug, the minute traces may not be detectable by these means because of the time lag between ingestion and collection of the sample.

Paper chromatography procedures are simple but cumbersome and lengthy. The standardisation of the atmosphere around the paper and vapour equilibrium in the chamber are vital and the entire procedure has to be mastered by running various controls and establishing the Rf values of one's own laboratory. Thin-Layer Chromatography is a good screening procedure but quantification of separated components is difficult. Gas Liquid Chromatography is useful for certain volatile substances like ethanol while HPLC is a highly sensitive, precise and accurate method. However, it is costly and requires good infrastructure and expertise. Immunoassay kits are being manufactured and provided by some reliable companies. These are used in many hospitals to monitor the therapeutic levels of some drugs like barbiturates and anti-epileptics. More kits are in the offing. These kits are simple to use and can be tested in an ordinary clinical chemistry laboratory.

When specimens of tissue, blood, urine, etc. are retrieved from fatal aircraft accident sites, the samples may be in a state of partial decomposition and desiccation. Whether any of these methods will succeed in such circumstances is a moot point. It is worthwhile to study this aspect by preparing experimental biological samples with known quantities of drugs of various groups, exposing them to vagaries of weather to cause partial decomposition/desiccation, etc. and then ascertaining the presence of drugs by various methods. This will give us an insight into the problem and if it is found that no method is suitable or worthwhile to detect the trace elements of drugs in decomposed and dried biological samples, a great deal of futile effort will be saved.

References

1. Mason JK. *Aviation Accident Pathology.* 1st ed. London: Butterworths, 1962.
2. Stevens PJ. *Fatal Civil Aircraft Accidents.* Bristol: John Wright & Sons, 1970.
3. Gilson JC, Stewart WK and Pekarek Z. Prevention of Injury in Aircraft Crashes. Flying Personnel Research Committee (FPRC) 556, Air Ministry, London, 1943; 556.
4. Hass GM. *Journal of Aviation Medicine* 1944; 15:77.
5. Teare D. Postmortem examinations on aircraft victims. *British Medical Journal* 1951; 2: 707.
6. Armstrong JA, Fryer DI, Stewart WA, Whittingham HE. Interpretation of Injuries in the Comet Aircraft Disasters. *Lancet* 1955; 1:1135–44.
7. Reals WJ. In Reals WJ ed. Medical Investigation of Aviation Accidents. Chicago Illinois: College of American Pathologists 1968; 2–4.
8. Hill IR. The Historical Background to Aerospace Pathology. *Aviation, Space and Environmental Medicine* 1982; 53(1):1–5.
9. Anderson IH. Aeromedical investigation of fatal aircraft accidents. *Aerospace Medicine* 1968; 39: 617–18.
10. Lovell FW, McMicheal H, Townsend FM. Pathology as an aid to reconstruction of aircraft accident. *Aerospace Medicine* 1960; 31: 745–48.
11. Townsend FM, Davidson WH, Hoyle BC. Two years' experience in combined engineering and pathology investigation in aircraft accidents. *Aerospace Medicine* 1962; 33: 913–19.
12. Adaval SK, Gandhi GS, Kunzru GN. An Analysis of Autopsy Investigations at IAM (1972–1976). *Aviation Medicine* 1979; 23: 96–102.
13. Townsend FM, Stembridge VA. Modern concepts in investigation of aircraft fatalities. *The Journal of Forensic Sciences* 1958; 3: 381–400.

14. Silliphant WM, Stembridge VA. The Role of pathologist in investigating aircraft accident fatalities. *US Forces Medical Journal* 1958; 9: 207.

15. Niess OK, Lentz EC, Townsend FM, Davidson WH, Chubb RM. The role of Physician in the investigation of aircraft accidents. *The Journal of the American Medical Association* 1963; 184: 701–4.

16. Editorial Comment. *British Medical Journal* 1964; 1:8.

17. Platt DS, Townsend FM. The function of the Pathologist in Aircraft Accident. *The Journal of Trauma* 1963; 3: 312–16.

18. Mason JK, Tarlton SW. Medical Investigation of the Loss of the Comet 4B Aircraft, 1967. *Lancet* 1967; 1: 431–34.

19. Gable WD. Pathology Patterns in Aircraft Accident Investigation. *Aerospace Medicine* 1968; 2: 638–40.

20. Townsend FM. The utilization of Pathology in Aircraft Accident Investigation. Medical aspects of flight safety. AFARDO graph 30 1959; 165–73. cited by Mason J.K. 1962.

21. Townsend FM. Medical Aspects of Aircraft Accidents. *Aerospace Medicine* 2nd ed. Randel HW. The William & Wilkins Co Ltd 1971; 310.

22. Berry FB. Icarus and the Physician, Reflections on Aircraft Accidents and their Prevention. *Journal of Aviation Medicine* 1956; 27: 197.

23. Cullen SA, Drysdale HC, Mayes RW. Role of Medical Factors in 1000 Fatal Aviation Accidents: Case Note Study. *British Medical Journal* 1997; 314: 1592.

24. Adaval SK, Kunzru GN, Verma RN. Pulmonary Fat Embolism in Aircrew Fatalities. *Aviation Medicine* 1980; 24(10): 6–8.

25. Kunzru GN, Adaval SK, Verma RN. Current Status of Fatal Aircraft Accident Investigation. *Aviation Medicine* 1979; 23: 129–31.

26. Indian Air Publication. Aircraft Accident Investigation and Prevention — a Guide to Medical Officers. *IAP* 4305 of 1978. Air Headquarters, New Delhi; 2:21.

27. Townsend FM. *Journal of Aviation Medicine* 1957; 28: 461.

28. Townsend FM. Pathologic Investigation of Aircraft Accident Fatalities. *Journal of Aviation Medicine* 1959; 28: 461.

29. Mason JK. Acute Coronary Insufficiency while at the controls of an aircraft: a report of two cases. *Medicine, Science and the Law* 1963; 3:194.

30. Mason JK. Asymptomatic Disease of Coronary Arteries in Young Men. *British Medical Journal* 1963; 2: 1234.

31. Jokl E, Mc Clellan JT. Sudden Cardiac Death of Pilots in Flight. *Cardiology* 1968; 52(4): 210–34.

32. Posey DM. Aerospace Pathology for the Flight Surgeon. Armed Forces Institute

of Pathology, Washington DC 1987.

33. Hellerich P, Pollak S. Airplane crash. Traumatological findings in cases of extreme body disintegration. *The American Journal of Forensic Medicine and Pathology* 1995; 16(4): 320–4.

34. Stevens L Cogswell. Aviation Pathology. *USAF Flight Surgeon's Guide* 1987; 15: 1–25.

35. Lichtenstein JD et al. Role of Radiology in Aviation Accident Investigation. *Aviation, Space and Environmental Medicine* 1980; 51: 1004.

36. Frank W Kiel, Blumberg M. Survey of Rotary Wing Aircraft Accidents. *Aerospace Medicine* 1963; 34(1): 42–7.

37. Pretre R, Murith N, Faidutti B. Increased association of cardiac and thoracic vascular lesions after closed trauma of the thorax. *Annals of Chirurgery* 1995; 49(9): 854–7.

38. Kunzru GN, Adaval SK. Aviation Pathological Evaluation of Fatal Aircraft Accidents Associated with Fire. *Journal of the Aeromedical Society of India* 1972; 15: 51–62.

39. Birky MM. The use of Soot Analysis as an investigative tool in aircraft fires. *Aviation, Space and Environmental Medicine*1989; 60: 72–7.

40. Krefft S. Who was at the aircraft's controls when the fatal accident occurred? *Aerospace Medicine* 1970; 41(7): 785–89.

41. Krefft S. Estimation of pilot control at the time of the crash. In Mason JK, Reals WJ (eds.). Aerospace Pathology, Chicago: College of American Pathologists' Foundation 1973.

42. Brownson P, Rowles JM, Wallace WA, Anton DJ. The mechanism of femoral fracture in an impact accident. *Aviation, Space and Environmental Medicine* 1998; 69(10): 971–4.

43. Mann RW, Holland TD. Perimortem calcaneal and talar fractures sustained in a military air crash in Vietnam. *Journal of the American Podiatric Medical Association* 1998; 88(9): 446–50.

44. Barwood AJ. Patterns of Ejection Injury. Joint Committee on Aviation Pathology, Seventh Scientific Session, Oct 1969. Royal Air Force Institute of Aviation Medicine UK.

45. Ekeland A. Injuries in military parachuting: a prospective study of 4499 jumps. *Injury* 1997; 28(3): 219–22.

46. Bar-Dayan Y, Shemer J. Parachuting injuries: a Retrospective Study of 43,542 Military Jumps. *Military Medicine* 1998; 163(1): 1–2.

47. Collin R, McCarthy GW, Kaleps I, Knox FS. Review of Major Injuries and Fatalities in USAF Ejections, 1981–1995. *Biomedical Science and Instrumentation* 1997; 33: 350–3.

48. Latham F, Howard P. Mechanisms of injury during Whole Body Linear Deceleration. Joint Committee on Aviation Pathology International symposium, Sep 1958.

49. Lillehei KO. A critical analysis of fatal injuries resulting from the Continental Flight 713 Airline Disaster: Evidence in favour of improved passenger restraint system. *Journal of Trauma* 1994; 37(5): 826–30.

50. Li G, Baker SP. Injury pattern in aviation-related fatalities. Implications for preventive strategies. *The American Journal of Forensic Medicine and Pathology* 1997; 18(3): 265–70.

51. Li G, Baker SP. Correlates of pilot fatality in general aviation crashes. *Aviation, Space and Environmental Medicine* 1999; 70(4): 305–9.

52. Reals WJ, Davidson WH, Karnitschnig HH. Pathology of light-aircraft accidents. *Aerospace Medicine* 1964; Feb: 133–5.

53. Mathur UB, Bannerjee B. An analysis of injuries in fatal aircraft accidents in Indian Air Force. *Indian Journal of Aerospace Medicine* 1988; 32(1): 32–40.

54. Dulchavsky SA, Geller ER, Iorio DA. Analysis of injuries following the crash of Avianca Flight 52. *Journal of Trauma* 1993; 34(2): 282–4.

55. McMeekin RR. Patterns of injury in fatal aircraft accidents. In Mason JK, Reals WJ (eds.). Aerospace Pathology. College of American Pathologists' Foundation, Chicago 1973.

56. Salomone J 3rd, Sohn AP, Ritzlin R, Gauthier JH, McCartty V. Correlations of injury, toxicology and cause of death to Galaxy Flight 203 crash site. *The Journal of Forensic Science* 1987 Sep; 32(5): 1403–15.

57. Modi NJ. *20th ed. Modi's Text Book of Medical Jurisprudence and Toxicology.* Tripathi Private Ltd Bombay 1977; 651.

58. Anderson WAD. Pathology. St Louis. The CV Mosby Co. 1977.

59. Adaval SK, Kunzru GN, Verma RN. Assessment of burns in accident fatalities. *Aviation Medicine* 1979; 23(2): 14–8.

60. Blackmore DJ. Interpretation of Carboxyhaemoglobin found at postmortem in victims of aircraft accidents. *Aerospace Medicine* 1970; 41(7): 759.

61. Glantz WM, Domienguez AM, Goldbaum LR, Christensen HE, Lovell FW, Gleason TL. Carbon Monoxide determination in aircraft accident fatalities. *Aerospace Medicine* 1959; 30: 711.

62. Mitchelnson BP. The Electron Energy-loss Spectroscopic Analysis of inhaled smoke particles. *Journal of Microscopy* 1992; 166(Pt 3): 381–7.

63. Chaturvedi AK. Aircraft fires, smoke toxicity and survival. *Aviation, Space and Environmental Medicine* 1996; 67(3): 275–8.

64. Dunne MJ, Jr, McMeekin RR. Medical investigation of fatalities from aircraft

accident burns. *Aviation, Space and Environmental Medicine* 1977; 48(10): 964–8.

65. Thompson RL. Cause of death in aircraft accidents: Drowning vs. traumatic injuries. *Aviation, Space and Environmental Medicine* 1977; 48(10): 924–8.

66. Gregersen M, Knudsen PJ, Jensen S. The crash of Partnair Convair 340/580 in the Skagerrak: traumatological aspects. *Aviation, Space and Environmental Medicine* 1995; 66(2):152–7.

67. White BD, Firth JL, Rowles JM. The effects of structural failure on injuries sustained in the MI Boeing 737 disaster, January 1989. NLDB Study Group. *Aviation, Space and Environmental Medicine* 1993; 64(2): 95–102.

68. McMeekin RR. Aircraft Accident Investigation. In Deltart RL (ed) *Fundamentals of Aerospace Medicine.* Philadelphia: Lea Febiger, 1985.

69. McCarty VO, Sohn AP, Ritzin RS, Gauthier JH. Scene investigation, identification and victim examination following the accident of Galaxy 203: Disaster preplanning does Work. *The Journal of Forensic Sciences* 1987 Jul; 32(4): 983–7.

70. Stevens PJ. Practical problems arising in the investigation of airline disasters abroad. *Aerospace Medicine* 1965; 36(7): 641–6.

71. Stevens PJ. Identification in Aviation Pathology. *Military Medicine* 1965; July: 653–61.

72. Cullen SA, Turk EP. The value of postmortem examination of passengers in fatal aviation accidents. *Aviation, Space and Environmental Medicine* 1980; 51(Pt 2): 1071–3.

73. Vidyasagar HRE, Devaiah MP, Murthy VSR. Analysis of Bird Strike Incidents of Fighter Aircraft (1975–86). Indian Air Force ADA/WB8/TR/001 Aeronautical Development Agency Bangalore (India) September 1986.

74. Defusco RP. 1987 Air Force Bird Strike Report. *USAF Flying Safety Magazine* 1988; 40(8): 2–5.

75. Mathur UB, Adaval SK. Laboratory Study on Avian Blood under Simulated Crash Conditions. *Indian Journal of Aerospace Medicine* 1993; 37(2):1–5.

76. Thomas FA. The Great Bird Detectives. *USAF Flying Safety Magazine* 1986; 42(10): 4–5.

77. Stork EJ. Urea Nitrogen-Uric Acid Ratio as a means of identifying avian tissue. *Aerospace Medicine* 1972; 43(2):172–5.

78. Bird. *The New Encyclopedia Britannica Macropaedia Vol. 2* Knowledge in depth. Hemingway Beuton.(15th edn.) Mc Graw Hill, London/Toronto 1981; 1953.

79. Sibley G, Ahlquest JE. Reconstructing Bird Phylogeny by comparing DNAs. *Scientific American* 1986; 254(2): 82–92.

80. Oser BL. Blood and other body fluids, In Hawk's *Physiological Chemistry.*

McGraw Hill Book Company. 14th ed. 14 1965; Chapter 12: 327–57.

81. Modi NJ. Examination of Blood Stain. *Modi's Text Book of Medical Jurisprudence and Toxicology*. Bombay, NM Tripathi Private Ltd. Ed. 20,1977; 95.

82. Flynn FV, Mayo P De. *Lancet* 1951; 261:235.

83. Schultz J, Grannis GF, Kimmel HB, Shay H. Federation Proc. 13(1954):131 as quoted by Riberio LP, Mietidien EE, Affonso OR in Paper Electrophoresis. A Review of Methods and Results. Elsevier Publishing Co. London/New York/Prinecton 1961; Chapter 17: 319.

84. La Ham QN. Report on aircraft turbine engine bird strike investigation. NRC Associate Committee on bird hazards to aircraft, Canada, 1967; Field Note No. 43, 17 Jan.

85. Petty AE, McMeekin RR. Laboratory examination of unidentified tissue fragments found at aircraft sites. *Aviation, Space and Environmental Medicine* 1977; 937–43.

86. Adaval SK, Kunzru GN. Histopathological findings in Reconstruction of Fatal Aircraft Accidents. *International Review of the Army, Navy and Air Force Medical Services* 1977; 11: 815–22.

87. Mason JK, Townsend FM, Jackson JR. *Aerospace Medicine* 1963; 34: 858.

88. Buley LE. *Aerospace Medicine* 1969; 40: 64.

89. Glantz WM, Stembridge VA. Coronary Artery Atherosclerosis as a factor in aircraft accident fatalities. *Journal of Aviation Medicine* 1959;30: 75.

90. Townsend FM, Glantz HG. Physiological training-officer. Paper presented at Annual Symposium, Alabama 1959 cited by Mason JK 1962.

91. Rayman RB. *Aerospace Medicine* 1974; 45: 86.

92. Adaval SK, Kunzru GN, Diwan RN, Verma RN. A Histological Study of Coronary Arteries in Aircrew Fatalities during 1962–1978. *Aviation Medicine* 1981; 25(1):1–6.

93. Tunstall Pedoe H. Risk of a Coronary Heart Attack in the normal population and how it might be modified in flyers. *The European Heart Journal* 1984; 5: 43–9.

94. Fechner GG, Sivaloganathan S. Demonstration of myocardial infarction in putrefying bodies. *Journal of Clinical Pathology* 1987; 40: 922–9.

95. Scheinman HZ. Coranary atherosclerosis in military pilots. Relationship to flying and aviation accidents, *Aerospace Medicine* 1968; 39: 1348.

96. Adaval SK, Akhtar M, Kunzru GN. Focal Myocarditis in a pilot involved in a Fatal Aircraft Accident. *Aviation Medicine* 1976; 19(2): 12–4.

97. Saphir O. Myocarditis: General Review with Analysis of 240 Cases. *Archives of Pathology* 1942; 33: 88.

98. Stevens PJ, Underwood Ground GKE. Occurrence and Significance of Myocarditis in trauma. *Aerospace Medicine* 1970; 46: 776.

99. Corby C. Isolated Myocarditis as a cause of sudden obscure death. *Medicine, Science and the Law* 1960; 1: 23.

100. Gormsen H. Sudden Unexplained Death due to Myocarditis. *Acta Pathologica et Microbiologica Scandinavia* 1955; 105–30.

101. Sopher IM. Myocarditis and the aircraft accidents. *Aerospace Medicine 1976; 45:963*

102. Warthin AS. Traumatic lipaemic and fatty embolism 171-227. *International Clinics* 1913; (Series), 23:171.

103. Lehman EP, Moore RN. Fat Embolism including experimental production without trauma. *Archives of Surgery* 1927; 14: 621.

104. Gauss H. The Pathology of Fat Embolism. *Archives of Surgery* 1924; 9: 592.

105. Denman FR, Gragg J. Fat Embolism: Diagnostic Enigma. *Archives of Surgery* 1948; 57: 325.

106. Robb Smith AHT. Pulmonary Fat Embolism. *Lancet* 1941; 1:135.

107. Vance BM. The Significance of Fat Embolism. *The American Journal of Pathology* 1931; 23: 426.

108. Warren S. Fat Embolism. *The American Journal of Pathology* 1946; 22: 69.

109. Wyatt JP, Khoo P. Fat Embolism in Trauma. *American Journal of Clinical Pathology* 1950; 20: 637.

110. Scully RE. Fat embolism in Korean Battle Casualties: its Incidence, Clinical Significance and Pathological Aspects. *The American Journal of Pathology* 1956; 32: 379.

111. Hickey JL, Stembridge VA. Occurrence of pulmonary fat and tissue embolism in aircraft accident fatalities. *Journal of Aviation Medicine* 1958; 29: 787.

112. Mason JK. Pulmonary Fat and Bone Marrow Embolism as an indication of ante mortem violence. *Medicine, Science and the Law* 1968; 8: 200.

113. Mason JK. *The Pathology of Violent Injury.* London, Edward Arnold 1978; Chapter 20.

114. Buchnan D, Mason JK. Occurrence of Pulmonary Fat and Bone Marrow Embolism. *The American Journal of Forensic Medicine and Pathology* 1982; 3(1): 73–8.

115. Busuttil A, Hanley JJ. A semi-automated micro-method for the histological assessment of fat embolism. *International Journal of Legal Medicine* 1994; 107(2): 90–5.

116. Bierre AR, Koelmeyer TD. Pulmonary fat and bone marrow embolism in aircraft accident victims. *Pathology* 1983; 15(2): 131–5.

117. Smith PW, Lacefield DJ, Grane CR. Toxicological findings in aircraft accident investigation. *Aerospace Medicine* 1970; 41(7): 760–2.

118. Anthony AT. Toxicology of aerospace systems. *Aerospace Medicine* 2nd ed. Ed. Randel HW. The William & Wilkins Co. Ltd 1971; 270.

119. Kunzru GN. Toxicology in Fatal Aircraft Accident Investigations. *Aviation Medicine* 1975; 19(2): 23.

120. Kuhlman JJ Jr, Levine B, Smith ML, Hordinsky JR. Toxicological Findings in Federal Aviation Administration general aviation accidents. *The Journal of Forensic Science* 1991; 36(4):1121–8.

121. Kapur RR, Adaval SK, Kunzru GN. Carbon Monoxide Toxicity in Fatal Aircraft Accident: A case report. *Aviation Medicine* 1977; 21: 82–5.

122. Blackmore DJ. *Aircraft Accident Toxicology: UK Experience* 1967–1972 cited in Carbon Monoxide (2nd edn.) EHC 1999; 213.

123. Dille JR, Linder MK. The Effects of Tobacco and Aviation Safety. *Aviation, Space and Environmental Medicine* 1981; 52(2): 112–5.

124. Goldbaum LR, Ramirez TG, Absalon KB. Joint Committee on Aviation Pathology XIII. What is the mechanism of carbon monoxide toxicity? *Aviation, Space and Environmental Medicine* 1975; 46(10):1289.

125. Goldbaum LR, Orellano T, Dergal E. Studies on the relation between Carboxyhaemoglobin Concentration and toxicity. *Aviation, Space and Environmental Medicine* 1977; 48: 969–972.

126. Adaval SK, Diwan RN. *Carboxyhaemoglobin in Preserved Blood Samples with Special Reference to Fatal Aircraft Accidents.* Armed Forces Medical Research Project No. 1270/81, 1981. Office of the Director General Armed Forces Medical Services, Government of India, Ministry of Defence, New Delhi.

127. Wayne EJ. Alcohol and Road Traffic. Proceedings of 3rd International Conference 1962; 118.

128. Froentjes W. In *Alcohol and Road Traffic.* London Butterworths1963; p 179.

129. Payne JP, Poster DV, Hill DW, Wood DGL. Observation on interpretation of blood alcohol level derived from analysis of urine. *British Medical Journal* 1967; 3: 819–23.

130. Payne JP, Hill DW, King NW. Observation on the distribution of alcohol in blood, breath and urine. *British Medical Journal* 1966; 1: 196–202.

131. Walls HJ. Urine Alcohol Tests and In-charge: Survey of 312 cases. *British Medical Journal* 1958; 21: 442.

132. Bennion J, Lynn Ting-kai Li. Alcohol retabolism in American Indians and Whites — Lack of racial differences in Metabolic Rate and Liver Alcohol Dehydrogenase. *The New England Journal of Medicine* 1976; 294(1): 9–13.

133. Kumar V, Adaval SK, Rai Kuldeep. After-effects of Alcohol on Psycho-physiological Functions in Relation to Flying Performance of Aircrew. Armed Forces Medical Research Project No. 423/71, 1971. Office of the Director General of Armed Forces Medical Services, Government of India, Ministry of Defence, New Delhi

134. Adaval SK, Maruthi Ram NK. A Comparative Study of Blood and Urine Ethanol Levels. *Aviation Medicine* 1977; 21: 31–4.

135. Todd-Sanford in Clinical Diagnosis by Laboratory Methods. Ed. Davidsohn & Henry. 15th ed., WB Saunders Co. 1980; Chapter 10:667–70.

136. Canfield DV, Kupiec T, Huffine E. Postmortem alcohol production in fatal aircraft accident. *The Journal of Forensic Sciences* 1993; 38(4): 914–7.

137. Kalant H. Interpretation of post-mortem ethanol concentrations. *Aerospace Medicine* 1968; 39: 633–7.

138. Johnson R, Lewis R, Canfield D, Dubowski K, Blank C. Utilizing the Urinary 5-HTOL/5-HIAA Ratio to Determine Ethanol Origin in Civil Aviation Accident victims. *The Journal of Forensic Sciences* 2005; 50(3).

139. Clinical Diagnosis and Management by Laboratory Methods by Todd, Sanford, Davidsohn. 17th ed. WB Saunders Co 1986.

140. Toxicology. Mechanisms and Analytical Methods. Edited by Stewart & Stoleman. Academic Press, NY 1961 Vol II:134–6.

141. Curry AS, Walker GW, Simpson GS. Estimation of ethanol in tissues and body fluids by Gas Chromatography. *Analyst* 1966; 91:1083.

142. Gradwohl's Clinical Laboratory Methods and Diagnosis. Edited by Sonnanwirth Leonard Jarett. 8th ed. 8, 1980; 406–9.

143. Gradwohl's Legal Medicine. Eds. Francis E Camps. 2nd ed., Bristol John Wright & Sons Ltd. 1968; 579.

144. *Aviation Medicine.* Edited by Geoffrey Dhenin. Tri-Med Books Ltd. London 1978; 11:149–51.

145. Adaval SK. Correlation of Blood and Breath Alcohol Levels with Task Performance. *Aviation Medicine* 1984; 28: 49–53.

146. Ryan LC, Mohler SR. Current role of alcohol as a factor in civil aircraft accidents. *Aviation, Space and Environmental Medicine* 1979; 50(3): 275–9.

147. Brown TC, Lane LC. Postmortem blood alcohol in general aviation pilots. *Aviation, Space and Environmental Medicine* 1977; 48(8): 771–5.

148. Harper CR, Albers WR. Alcohol and General Aviation Accidents. *Aerospace Medicine* 1964; 35: 462.

149. Asksnes EN. Effects of small doses of alcohol upon performance in a Link Trainer. *Journal of Aviation Medicine* 1954; 25: 680–8.

150. Billing CE, Wick RL, Gerke RJ, Chase RC. Effects of Ethyl Alcohol on Pilot Performance. *Aerospace Medicine* 1973; 379–82.

151. Henry PH, Fluech JA, Sanford JF, Keiser HN, McNee RC, Walter WH, Webster KH, Hartman BO, Lancaster MC. Assessment of performance in a Link GAT-1 Flight Simulator at three alcohol dose levels. *Aerospace Medicine* 1974; 45: 33–44.

152. Harper CP, William AL. Alcohol and General Aviation Accidents. *Aerospace Medicine* 1964; 35(5): 462–4.

153. Mohler SR, Berner WH, Goldbaum LR. Alcohol question in Aircraft Accident Investigation. *Aerospace Medicine* 1968; 39: 1228–30.

154. Mohler SR. *Civil Aviation Medicine* 2nd ed. Randel HW. The William & Wilkins Co. Ltd. 1971: 647.

155. Ryan LC, Mohler SR. Intoxicating Liquor and General Aviation Pilot in 1971. *Aerospace Medicine* 1972; 43(9): 1024–6.

156. Alha AR, Tamminen V. Detection of alcohol in aviation and other fatalities in Finland. *Aerospace Medicine* 1971; 42(5): 564–8.

157. Davis GL. Alcohol and Military Aviation Fatalities. *Aerospace Medicine* 1968; 39: 869–72.

158. Davis GL. Postmortem Alcohol Analysis of General Pilot Fatalities, AFIP 1962–1967. *Aerospace Medicine* 1973; 44(1): 80–3.

159. Zeller AF. Alcohol and other drugs in Aircraft Accidents. *Aviation, Space and Environmental Medicine* 1975; 46: 1271–4.

160. Cook CC. Alcohol and Aviation. *Addiction* 1997; 92(5): 539–55.

161. Blackmore DJ. The detection of drugs at therapeutic concentrations as applied to Aviation Toxicology. *The Journal of Forensic Sciences* 1969; 14(4): 545–54.

162. Chaturvedi AK, Canfield DV. Role of Metabolites in Aviation Forensic Toxicology. *Aviation, Space and Environmental Medicine* 1997; 68(3): 230–3.

163. Akin A, Chaturvedi AK. Selective Serotonin Reuptake Inhibitors in Pilot Fatalities of Civil Aviation Accidents, 1990–2001. *Aviation, Space and Environmental Medicine* 2003; 74(11): 1169–76.

164. Clark EGC. Isolation and Identification of Drugs. Ed. Clarke EGC. London. The Pharmaceutical Press 1969; 1.

165. Recent Advances in Clinical Biochemistry. Ed. Alberti KGMM. New York. Churchill Livingstone 1978; 1.

Index